The Political Economy of Developmental Disabilities

The Political Economy of Developmental Disabilities

by
Paul J. Castellani, Ph.D.
Director
Program Research
New York State Office of Mental Retardation
and Developmental Disabilities
Albany

·P·A·U·L·H·
BROOKES
PUBLISHING CO.

Baltimore · London

Paul H. Brookes Publishing Co.
Post Office Box 10624
Baltimore, MD 21285-0624

Copyright © 1987 by Paul H. Brookes Publishing Co., Inc.
All rights reserved.

Typeset by The Composing Room, Grand Rapids, Michigan.
Manufactured in the United States of America by
Thomson-Shore, Inc., Dexter, Michigan.

Library of Congress Cataloging-in-Publication Data
Castellani, Paul J., 1942–
    The political economy of developmental disabilities.

    Bibliography: p.
    Includes index.
    1. Developmentally disabled—Services for—United
States.   2. Developmentally disabled—Government
policy—United States.   I. Title
HV3006.A4C37   1987   362.1′968   86-26409
ISBN 0-933716-79-6

Contents

Preface

MOST OF THE INFORMATION CONTAINED IN THIS BOOK IS WELL UNDERSTOOD BY A large number of people in administrative, policy-making, and operational roles in developmental services, in both the private and public sectors. In fact, I first became aware of the complexity of the issues of public and private finance and the capacity of local officials and agency executives to manage in the rapidly changing world of developmental services from informal discussions with these individuals that were conducted in the context of more formal research projects. Later, I was able to check back to the literature, to government officials in Albany and Washington, and to sources in other states to verify this information and to place it in the appropriate framework, thereby adding building materials to the basic structure. Most of these individuals have had neither the time nor the inclination to make their observations known to a broader field of policy-makers and analysts; therefore, in many respects, this book is intended to be a bridge for carrying their insights to that broader audience.

A book that uses "political economy" in the title is not entirely a grassroots endeavor. (Actually, in Chapter 1, the rather straightforward "interdependence between political and economic processes" meaning of that term is explained.) Nonetheless, many of the problems that arise at the point of delivery—the community context of services—are new, complex, and ambiguous. Moreover, the dynamics of finance, organization of services, selection of clients, and policy-making often seem to be either unrelated or perversely related. This book attempts to place those problems and issues in a coherent framework that helps us make sense of that confusing world, and enhances our ability to solve these problems. Many of the central concerns facing all human services and the social sciences in general are those that are at the core of the experience in the field of developmental disabilities. However, it also seems that the benefits of this experience have not always been adequately translated to other arenas, nor have we taken full advantage of some of the perspectives and approaches of political science and economics. This book is also a "pracademic's" attempt to bridge theory and practice so that contributions are made to both arenas.

Of course, thinking about a project like this and actually doing it are two entirely different things. Writing this book required a lot of help from friends, colleagues, and the individuals who are in those policy-making, service delivery, administrative, and other roles where the central issues addressed in this book are actually being played out.

In addition to those insights gleaned from a wide variety of sources over the past few years, a number of people were interviewed specifically for this book. Those interviews were conducted with the understanding that no one would be specifically identified in the text, but their comments and observations were critical to describing the dynamics of community-based services. Those people include Margery Ames, James Ansley, Marc Brandt, Michael Fox, Joni Fritz, Joel Levy, Michael Morris, Michael Reif, and Alfred Tuttle.

John Agosta, Melissa Behm, David Braddock, Ronald Conley, Robert Gettings, John Gargan, Martin Hanlon, Bernard Humphrey, John Noble, and Colleen Wieck were especially helpful in reading drafts, suggesting changes, and providing me with a wealth of information from their experience and knowledge in the field.

The support and advice of Paul Puccio and my colleagues in Program Research have been crucial to completing this project. William Bird, in particular, has made an extraordinary contribution to the book.

Most importantly, Donna Castellani has gotten me through the hard parts with her patience and understanding.

The Political Economy of Developmental Disabilities

1

Introduction

THIS BOOK IS ABOUT POWER AND MONEY. ITS BASIC PREMISE IS THAT THE amount of developmental services in communities, the ways in which those services are provided and organized, who receives those services, and how their costs are allocated and their benefits distributed are the outcomes of political and economic processes.

There are millions of people with developmental disabilities in this country, and the financial cost to the public of providing them care and services is a significant component of human services budgets. The direct private financial costs to these individuals, their families, and society are enormous as well. The field of developmental disabilities not only encompasses substantial public and private endeavors but also there have been changes in this arena over the past 10 to 15 years that have been virtually revolutionary when compared to other human services. New ways of thinking about the roles and place of people with developmental disabilities have formed the basis of a powerful political ideology. Aggressive advocacy for the rights of these people to lead a more normal life has resulted in federal and state policy initiatives that have brought about massive shifts in the locus of care of thousands of people and a shift in responsibility for care from state to the local levels of government. As complex arrays of developmental services have evolved in communities, a private sector has emerged and assumed a greater importance in the provision of care. Although these changes pose innumerable questions and problems, at one fundamental level they involve an enormous amount of political power and a great deal of public and private money.

The purpose of this book is three-fold: (1) to identify the central issues and problems in a new system of community-based developmental services, (2) to analyze the factors that affect the amounts of services that are available and the ways in which they are delivered, and (3) to examine those issues and problems in a political economy framework that shows the relationships among them and organizes them in a manner that enhances one's ability to resolve the emerging problems in this new policy arena.

THE CHANGING ENVIRONMENT
OF DEVELOPMENTAL SERVICES

The changes that have taken place in the field of developmental services have been numerous and substantial in almost all respects. The new circumstances that have been created require a new and expanded perspective on the nature of developmental services, who receives them, how they are delivered and organized, and the public and private processes that affect their availability and accessibility in communities.

The movement of large numbers of people with developmental disabilities from state-operated institutions to smaller residential and day programs in communities has been one of the most significant processes in contemporary social policy. At about the same time and in response to many of the same pressures, children with handicapping conditions have been provided free and appropriate education. In many respects these processes have not yet been fully implemented because many thousands of people remain in institutions, and all children with disabilities are not receiving a free and appropriate education. Advocates, analysts, and policy-makers are still focusing their energy on the public policy processes that address these problems. Moreover, the political and economic dynamics that are associated with these processes continue to have a significant impact on the size and shape of developmental services.

The success of deinstitutionalization and other efforts to establish community-based developmental services, although not yet complete, has created a significantly different set of problems and issues. Developmental services in community contexts involve new types of services, clients, providers, policy-making processes, and environmental factors that affect the outcomes that advocates, policy-makers, and other key actors expect to achieve. Merely recognizing these changes is not sufficient to address the problems that have arisen or to outline the features of a community-based system of services that is posited as the outcome of deinstitutionalization and the creation of developmental services in communities. Those key features must be identified and the significant factors that affect their size and shape be described.

The most obvious and yet problematic feature of the new environment of developmental services is that the entire context of services is changing. Tens of thousands of people have moved from being segregated from society, receiving no services if they lived at home, or being institutionalized in remote places, to living in communities, going to school, working, and receiving habilitative and support services from a variety of sources. Although advocates, policy-makers, and analysts talk about the *community* as the best context for people with developmental disabilities, it is obvious that communities are different. In fact, there seems to be an effort in the field to avoid defining what is a community. Nonetheless, it is important that those features of communities that are important to people with developmental disabilities be identified and their impact on community-based services be assessed.

The second major change that is occurring involves new types of people with developmental disabilities who are seeking access to services in communities. The definition of developmental disabilities has changed to encompass disabilities other than mental retardation and to use a functional rather than a categorical approach. Under the new definition, there are many unanswered questions about how many people might require services, how their needs for services should be assessed, and what the factors are that affect their need for or influence their access to community-based developmental services.

The services in community contexts are different in many respects from those in institutions. For a large number of people who have been deinstitutionalized, many of the same types of services are provided in separate settings or in relatively intensive models, such as intermediate care facilities for the mentally retarded (ICFs/MR). However, new types of services, such as family support services and independent living centers, are emerging that are unique to community settings. Moreover, there has been a very important shift from public to private provision of services for many people, and there are new types of agencies with various auspices and organizational structures providing services. The relationships among providers of developmental services and other human services agencies in communities are also undergoing significant changes. What are the factors that determine the ways developmental services are provided and organized, and what are the consequences for people with developmental disabilities? Most attention to the issues of service models has been rather narrowly focused on the attributes of specific program sites or services. Very little has been written about the attributes of developmental service systems and the ways that the organization of services relates to their availability and accessibility in communities.

The community context of developmental services involves substantially different public policy structures, processes, and issues. The process of deinstitutionalization, the mandates for education for all handicapped children, and the creation of most of the developmental services in communities have been the result of a variety of federal and state government policy processes. To this point the posture of most local governments has been reactive and negative. Nonetheless, if developmental services are to become a community-based system of services, then local governments must play a larger and more proactive role. The unique structures and processes of local government, as well as the problems and issues peculiar to this level of policy-making, need to be identified and their impact on developmental services assessed.

Community-based developmental services also involve a variety of public and private actors, interests, and activities. Over the past 15 years, virtually all the issues and problems affecting people with developmental disabilities have fallen within the public domain. People with developmental disabilities have been clients, their families advocates, their care the province of public institutions, and changes in these circumstances the result of federal and state public policies. Public policies still remain the center of attention. However, the new community context of services encompasses a broader range of actors and activities that are linked to the public sector but that also operate within a distinctly private environment. This environment not only includes private voluntary and proprietary service organizations but also includes employers, people with developmental disabilities who work, families who bear many of the costs of care, and communities that benefit economically from the provision of developmental services. An analysis of the features of a community-based system of developmental services must take into account the importance of private sector activities and relationships.

Finally, understanding the community context of services requires a more careful definition of the outcomes that are expected to be achieved through those policy processes and other activities. Deinstitutionalization is certainly not easily achieved, but the measurement of success is relatively straightforward. The success in establishing community-based services is somewhat more difficult to measure. Numbers of residential beds and day service slots are often used as measures of the availability of community-based services. However, many of the new types of services that are emerging in the community context are more intermittent and less well defined, and the measurement of their availability becomes more difficult. Community-based services are also expected to be accessible, but that is a concept that is even more troublesome as a measure of the effectiveness of a community-based system of services. Accessibility includes such characteristics of programs and services as location and cost, as well as eligibility criteria for entrance to services, and these latter eligibility aspects of accessibility are particularly difficult to assess. Moreover, accessibility carries with it a notion of appropriateness: access to a program or service that addresses the needs of the person with a developmental disability. Throughout this book, the phrase "availability and accessibility of community-based services" is used, but it is with the recognition that those terms are usually indicative of a very general set of goals.

In general, the community context of developmental services presents a substantially distinct set of issues and problems for the field of developmental disabilities. These problems have only recently emerged, and the factors that are important to the establishment of community-based developmental services systems are still unclear. One important objective of this book is to identify and describe the types of issues and problems in this new environment that are significant to the establishment of community-based service systems.

THE POLITICAL ECONOMY FRAMEWORK

The description of some of the most important dimensions of the new community context of services makes it clear that a cohesive and comprehensive framework for analysis of the issues and problems is required. At the minimum, a perspective within which the problems can be organized is needed. Political economy provides this framework and perspective.

In its most simple and straightforward form, political economy is concerned with understanding the relationships between politics and economics in a particular arena. There are a wide variety of schools of political economy that entail a number of distinct normative perspectives, proceed from either an economics or political science basis, and involve highly theoretical constructs and methodologies (Ilchman & Upoff, 1969; Lindblom, 1977; Schultze, 1985; Staniland, 1985). However, for many analysts, the political economy perspective is largely concerned with public policy, but also encompasses an assessment of the reciprocal relationships between economic and political processes; it does not entail a particular methodology (Staniland, 1985). It is this latter use of political economy that provides the framework of analysis for this book.

Within the political economy framework a number of factors that are emerging as significant in the community context of developmental services can be included. Labor costs, product marketing, the role of private proprietary firms in the delivery services, and the economic behavior of people with developmental disabilities, their families, and service organizations are only a few of the issues that have become important considerations and are readily encompassed within a political economy framework. In addition, economics, more than political science, readily provides an appreciation for some of the broader implications of public policy, or as put by one commentator, "You must remember that every dollar of expenditure is someone's dollar of income." Finally, the political economy framework is sensitive to the fact that not all the factors and activities affecting community-based developmental services fall within the public domain, and that private as well as public transactions must be taken into account. For example, individuals and families may purchase developmental services, insurance, and supportive services from a variety of private vendors, and the extent and nature of these market transactions are important to the understanding of community-based services. In summary, the political economy framework is used in this book to indicate the need to broaden the perspective to encompass both economic and political processes, to point to issues and problems that fall largely in the realm of economics, and to examine the relationships between the public and private sectors in considering the size and structure of developmental service systems.

The Political Systems Model

Although political economy is the overarching framework for considering both private and public elements of community-based services, these services are still largely within the public domain. Thus, the concepts inherent in the political systems model provide most of the operational guidelines to the processes and factors at work in this policy arena.

The political systems model associated most closely with David Easton (1957, 1965) is an approach that views public policy (outputs) as a response to forces (inputs) brought to bear on the political system from its environment. This model is especially useful because it requires that the linkages among the environment, the institutions of the political system, and those public policy outputs be taken into account. Figure 1.1 is a simplified diagram of the political systems model.

Institutions of the political system include interrelated legislative, judicial, and executive branches, and public bureaucracies at the federal, state, and local levels. It is particularly important to appreciate the fact that those relationships are multidimensional. Demands in the form of class action suits can be brought in federal

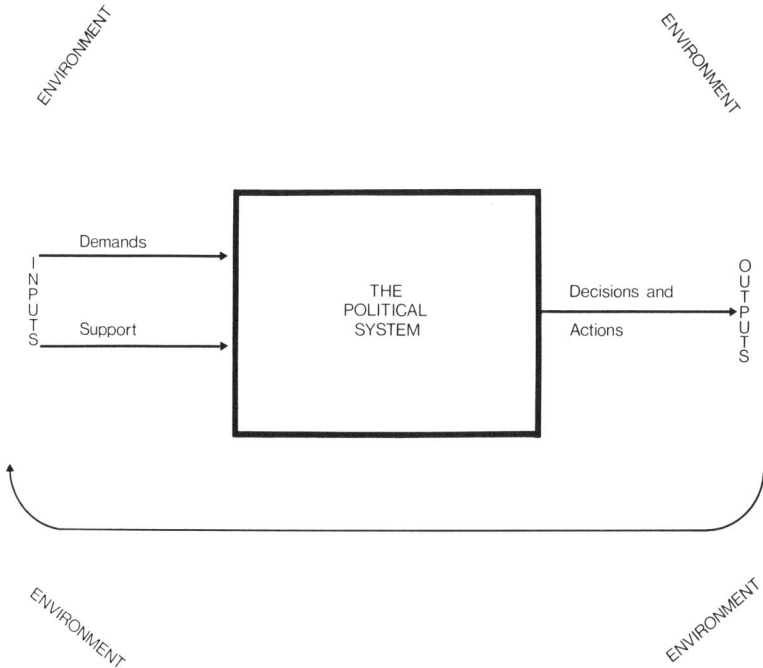

Figure 1.1. Political systems model.

courts to direct state government bureaucracies to effect deinstitutionalization, or a federal statute can require local school districts to
provide free and appropriate education to children with disabilities.
The political systems model forces the analyst of public policy to be
cognizant of the linkages that result in public policy and to be sensitive to the factors in the environment that give rise to demands
(inputs), as well as the outcomes of public policy in that environment. Those concepts and guidelines are important to the understanding of community-based services.

Political economy forms the framework of the book, and the
political systems model provides much of the language and operational guidelines for analysis of the public policies and private activities that are its focus. However, beyond any framework or analytic approach, a central objective of the book is to call attention to the
fact that politics and economics are central to the size and structure
of community-based services. To many professionals that may seem
self-evident. However, there also seems to be an inclination in the
field—and perhaps it is more widely shared—to view political and
economic considerations as necessary evils, or to assume incorrectly

that courts are insulated from political pressures, or to discount the values of legislators who are hostile to the goals of advocates. This book points out the linkages among political institutions and processes at all levels of government, their relationships to economic activities and the sociodemographic characteristics of the environment, and their collective impact on the policy outcomes of critical importance to the field of developmental disabilities. It argues that the interests of advocates, policy-makers, and analysts are best served by a broad-based analytic framework. Although power and money often have negative connotations, those forces are not necessarily bad if they are directed toward the positive goals of advocates and policy-makers. Available and accessible community-based developmental services are the outcomes of political and economic processes, and how those activities are related to those ends is the subject of this book.

PLAN OF THE BOOK

Community-based developmental services are the main focus of this book. The book examines the factors and processes that influence the amount of services and the ways in which they are provided, how they are funded, who receives services, and how the local policy environment affects the ways in which they are supported, managed, and coordinated.

In Chapter 2, the recent history of developmental services is reviewed because the dynamics of the large-scale changes that have taken place over the past 10 to 15 years in this area continue to exert a powerful influence on the evolution of community-based services. The political ideologies that provide agendas for advocates and guidelines for policy-makers, the components of the legal framework within which these changes have occurred, and the funding streams that have supported and shaped the structure of developmental services are the three dimensions along which this recent history is examined.

The economics of community-based services is the topic of Chapter 3. Public financing is the dominant economic factor in the field, and the sources, amounts, and types of funding for various programs are reviewed. However, several other significant economic factors that have not received adequate attention are explored and their linkages to public finance described. The economic behavior of individuals with disabilities and their families in the context of community services is analyzed, and the roles of such other key actors as employees of service agencies and those organizations themselves are described. Moreover, the impact of the community on developmental services and the reciprocal impact of developmental services on communities are also examined.

The question of who gains access to community-based services is the focus of Chapter 4. The chapter first examines some of the concepts of disability and how their application in other areas has relevance to the issue of who is developmentally disabled. That problem of definition is also considered in light of changes from categorical to functional definitions of developmental disabilities, as well as the epidemiologic problems involved. The major portion of the chapter explores the wide variety of situational, sociodemographic, and service system characteristics that influence who actually receives services in the community.

The organization of community-based developmental services is discussed in Chapter 5. Two major concerns are examined in this chapter. First, the various new kinds of services that have emerged in community contexts, as well as changes in traditional service models, are described and their implications examined. Second, organizations that provide developmental services are discussed, and the impact of various types, structures, and auspices on the availability and accessibility of services is described.

In Chapter 6, decision-making at the point of delivery—the community context of services—is examined. A brief historical review shows that responsibility for care of people with mental disabilities has shifted between state and local governments. Next, the various dimensions of the local capacity to support, provide, and manage developmental services are described. The particularly troublesome problems of governance at the local level and their impact on developmental services are discussed. Finally, the issues involved in the coordination and integration of developmental services are explored.

The final chapter of the book pulls together the major observations and conclusions from each chapter and indicates some of the problems and opportunities in the evolution of community-based developmental services.

2

The Impact of
The Recent History in
Developmental Disabilities
on The Future of
Community-Based Services

THE PREMISE OF THIS CHAPTER IS THAT THE SHAPE OF THE FUTURE IS determined to a great degree by the past. Therefore, a review of the recent history in this policy area should provide important information about the nature of current problems and the shape of future directions. This chapter also shows that, although the magnitude and directions of changes in services for people with developmental disabilities have been large and positive, cross-currents remain in the various dimensions of change that exert pressures that have a perplexing impact on the evolution of community-based services.

The creation of large numbers of community-based services within a relatively short period of time is related to a variety of public policy initiatives and proposals for reform. Federal court orders and consent decrees, the mandates of the 1975 Education for All Handicapped Children Act (PL 94-142) and other federal and state statutes, and new mechanisms for funding developmental services have all played a role in service development. New concepts about where and how people with developmental disabilities should be served have also made significant contributions to these changes.

In this chapter, these various proposals and policy initiatives are described along three broad dimensions: 1) the *political ideologies* that have defined the goals for advocates, shaped the political agenda, and provided the conceptual bases for policy directions in this area; 2) the *legal frameworks* that form the authoritative bases for changes in services; and 3) the *financing* of developmental ser-vices. A description of the changes along these three dimensions indicates the enormous impact that these proposals and initiatives collectively have had on services for people with developmental disabilities. This analysis also points to the incongruities among and within these proposals that continue to affect the availability and accessibility of community-based services.

POLITICAL IDEOLOGY: CIVIL RIGHTS, NORMALIZATION, AND THE LEAST RESTRICTIVE ALTERNATIVE

Americans typically view their politics as pragmatic and largely free of pronounced ideological content. It is indeed difficult to identify the social theory that underlies many of the policy initiatives advo-cated in various political arenas, and even such general labels as liberal or conservative (at least the former) are eschewed by elected officials. Nonetheless, it must be recognized that the policy goals pursued by advocates for change are at least implicitly informed with a political ideology: a more or less coherent source of guiding principles and justification for political action (Lowi, 1979).

The changes in the ways in which services are provided to peo-ple with developmental disabilities have been guided by a rather explicit political ideology. Indeed, three distinct strands in this po-litical ideology have been employed as rationalizations for reform and conceptual frameworks guiding advocates and policy-makers: 1) civil rights, 2) the principle of normalization, and 3) the principle of the least restrictive alternative. In this section of the chapter, the major elements of these three strands of the political ideology in this arena are described and their impact on the establishment of com-munity-based services assessed.

Civil Rights

It is difficult to separate the concept of civil rights as a component of a political ideology from the actual court cases in which those rights are sought and defined. Those cases of particular importance to the field of developmental disabilities arose from the civil rights move-ment; the application of the notion of civil rights to the circum-stances of people with developmental disabilities constitutes an important element of the political ideology in the area.

In the early 1960s, the impact of psychotropic drugs began to be felt in the mental health field. These so-called tranquilizing drugs were increasingly used to treat people with mental illness outside the confines of large state-operated psychiatric hospitals. This form of treatment provided the therapeutic underpinnings of the growth of community psychiatry.

The use of tranquilizing drugs and the development of a community perspective in the treatment of mentally ill people occurred at the same time that the civil rights movement was winning major legislative and judicial victories and altering public perceptions. Although the primary focus of the civil rights movement was to guarantee the rights of racial minorities, the association between civil rights and the conditions of individuals housed in state hospitals was soon made.

Studies of the conditions of patients in mental hospitals concluded that the civil rights of these individuals were abridged in a number of ways (Special Committee to Study Commitment Procedures, 1962). As a result of these reviews, some reforms in due process guarantees surrounding commitment procedures were undertaken through state statute (Castellani, 1975). At the same time the heightened sensitivity to the abridgement of the civil rights of patients in mental hospitals gave rise to a series of lawsuits in both federal and state courts that sought to redress those problems.

A series of decisions by state courts extended due process and habeas corpus guarantees to the criminally insane, to mentally ill defendants, and to people found not guilty by reason of insanity (Steadman & Cocozza, 1974). In New York State these decisions resulted in the transfer of several hundred mentally ill or similarly situated individuals from the state's prisons to state mental hospitals. (Hunt & Wiley, 1968). Most important, the federal courts, in cases involving the criminally insane, moved beyond procedural guarantees, such as due process, to substantive rights. In *Rouse v. Cameron* (1967) the Federal Court of Appeals gave a substantial impetus to the "right to treatment" principle, and in *Covington v. Harris* (1969) the federal court defined the "least restrictive alternative" principle.

The immediate outcomes of these decisions were the administrative actions noted above and the allocation of some additional funds to provide the more therapeutic services that the courts mandated (Castellani, 1975). Further, as a result of initiatives in the area of the rights of mental patients, the courts asserted themselves as activist decision-making structures. In doing so, they not only created a new and important role in state-level political processes but also established procedural and substantive civil rights that could be applied to other client groups in related circumstances. Thus, the changes that would be mandated through federal and state courts, as well as through statute, had the important concepts of civil rights as a rationale for change and a set of procedural guidelines and substantive outcomes to be achieved.

Principle of Normalization

The concepts of civil rights provided the ideological and operational bases for the court cases that produced much of the change in this area, particularly in the early stages of reform. At about the same time in the 1960s, the principle of normalization was being developed and articulated, and this central element of the political ideology formed an overarching rationale for deinstitutionalization and the creation of community-based services.

The principle of normalization has evolved over the years, but Lakin and Bruininks (1985) provide a definition that captures the essential features of the concept:

> This standard (normalization) dictates that the residential, educational, employment, and social and recreational conditions of the individual must be close to the cultural norm for a person of that age as the extent of the individual's disability reasonably allows. (p. 11)

Two of the most remarkable aspects of the principle of normalization are its relative newness and its almost immediate widespread acceptance throughout the field of developmental disabilities. The earliest uses of the term "normalization" are usually credited to Nirje (1969) and Bank-Mikkelson (1969). However, the term has become most closely associated with Wolf Wolfensberger and his associates through a large number of publications on the topic beginning in 1972 (Wolfensberger, 1972, 1983; Wolfensberger & Glenn, 1973; Wolfensberger & Tullman, 1982).

Indeed, the principle's rapid and widespread adoption throughout the field has both indicated normalization's power as a political ideology and brought a recent call for revision in its definition by Wolfensberger (1983). Wolfensberger argues that "once people hear or see the term 'normalization,' a large proportion (apparently even the vast majority) assume—usually wrongly—that they know 'what it means'" (p. 234). Wolfensberger goes on to propose that normalization be called "social role valorization." He does not provide as succinct a definition of either normalization or its proposed successor, social role valorization, as that offered by Lakin and Bruininks or a large number of others in the field who have found the term "normalization" to be a clear, succinct, widely understood, and almost universally agreed-upon guideline for political action. Without question, normalization is now at the core of the current political ideology in the field of developmental disabilities.

Least Restrictive Alternative

The principle of the least restrictive alternative operates with the principle of normalization as an exceptionally powerful element within the political ideology associated with deinstitutionalization and the development of community-based services for people with developmental disabilities. Lakin and Bruininks (1985) again provide a clear and succinct definition:

> In general, the policy of placing handicapped persons in the least restrictive environment means that developmentally appropriate care, training, and support based on an individual's needs should be, to the maximum extent possible, provided in the types of community settings that are used by nonhandicapped persons. (p. 13)

The principle of the least restrictive alternative was originally given a legal expression in the case of *Covington v. Harris* in 1969 and was applied to the status of mentally ill patients in correctional facilities. However, it has most recently been widely applied to people with developmental disabilities. It has been particularly important as a standard in legislation and judicial decisions affecting free and appropriate education for children with handicapping conditions (Bachrach, 1985; Lakin & Bruininks, 1985). Although the meaning and derivation of the term have been explored in some depth (Bachrach, 1985), the simplicity and virtual face validity of the concept have allowed it to be almost universally acknowledged throughout the field and adopted as a standard and guide for advocacy and political decision-making.

Implications of Political Ideology for Community-Based Services

As suggested above, it is extremely difficult to gauge the effect of political ideology on public policy. Nevertheless, even a cursory review of the field in the past 10 years indicates the prominence and widespread acceptance and expression in public policy of the concepts of civil rights and the principles of normalization and the least restrictive alternative. The following description of the changes in the legal framework of developmental services also indicates that these elements of the political ideology in this area have had a distinct and, in some respects, inconsistent impact on public policy outcomes. Although each of the major strands of the political ideology continues to exert an important influence, the overall paradigm has shifted.

LEGAL FRAMEWORK FOR
DEINSTITUTIONALIZATION
AND COMMUNITY-BASED SERVICES

Within the legal framework affecting the recent changes in deinstitu-tionalization and community-based services, the fundamental issue is authority. Advocacy for people with developmental disabilities has been organized in large measure around a philosophy of nor-malization that provides a set of goals and standards that measure their attainment. Indeed, within the definition of the political sys-tem, normalization forms the political ideology that shapes the de-mands made on the political system. The legal framework consists of the authoritative outputs of government that ultimately invoke the power of the state. There are a wide variety of authoritative outputs, but they typically include statutes, court decisions, and regulations at all levels of government. These constitute the legal framework; that is, the authoritative guidelines and parameters that have shaped deinstitutionalization and the establishment of community-based services.

Impact of Federal Court Decisions

For long periods of time in our history, the judicial system has had an important impact on people with mental disabilities (Deutsch, 1949). However, until the contemporary Warren Court in the 1950s, the courts functioned most often as instruments through which the police and *parens patriae* powers of the state were exercised (Castellani, 1975; Friedman & Daly, 1973; Szasz, 1963). The civil rights movement had an important effect on the care of people with mental disabilities by securing procedural and substantive rights for people in institutions. Initially, the rights that had been won for people with mental illness in institutions were sought for people with developmental disabilities also living in institutions. The shift from institutional guarantees to abolition of institutions through the courts is discussed in the context of the *Wyatt, Willowbrook,* and *Pennhurst* cases.

    Wyatt v. Stickney: The Right to Treatment During the 1960s the focus of parent group advocacy for people with developmental disabilities was generally on securing more services and improved conditions in new or renovated institutions (Castellani, Tausig, & Bird, 1984). However, advocacy through the federal court process began to take an important new direction with the *Wyatt v. Stickney* (1972) suit in Alabama.

Wyatt v. Stickney, which was brought against the Commissioner of Mental Health of Alabama, was a class action complaint on behalf of a resident of Bryce State Hospital for the mentally ill. The complaint had its genesis in the prospect of mass termination of employees at Bryce State Hospital and the consequential prospect of "no treatment," which prompted Federal Judge Johnson to invoke Rouse v. Cameron (1967) and the "right to treatment" provision of that decision. Subsequent to the initial order in the case, several national organizations, including the American Association on Mental Deficiency and the National Association for Retarded Citizens, joined the suit as amici curiae, and the complaint was amended to include the other state institution for the mentally ill and the state institution for the mentally retarded: Partlow State School and Hospital. (Castellani, 1975).

Although there were a number of interim actions and orders in the Wyatt case, the final order represented a major landmark in judicial policy-making in this area and public policy-making in general. The court found that the evidence "vividly and undisputedly" demonstrated that the conditions at Partlow did not meet constitutionally minimum standards. It also rejected the argument of the Alabama Mental Health Board that the absence of adequate funding precluded appropriate staffing and facilities. Judge Johnson stated that the implementation of constitutionally minimum standards was mandatory, and no default could be justified by a want of operating funds. The court went so far as to point out that, if the Alabama Legislature failed to provide sufficient funds to implement these standards, it would "take affirmative steps including the appointment of a master to ensure that proper funding is realized" (Wyatt v. Stickney, 1972). The court even suggested that a special session of the Alabama Legislature be held to appropriate the necessary funding, and it preferred the notion of seizing and selling state property to secure the funds if the legislature failed to act. The court also ordered the hiring of a "professionally qualified and experienced administrator" to oversee reform and reorganization at Partlow. Appendix A to the Final Order and Decree was "Minimum Constitutional Standards for Adequate Habilitation of the Mentally Retarded," and 49 detailed standards were stipulated covering: 1) Adequate Habilitation of Residents, 2) Individualized Habilitation Plans, 3) Humane Physical and Psychological Environment, and 4) Qualified Staff in Numbers Sufficient to Provide Adequate Habilitation.

The Wyatt v. Stickney case clearly established entire new dimensions in public policy with respect to institutionalized people with mental retardation. In the first instance it was a class action suit, and this type of suit later became a judicial vehicle to bring about large-scale change, affecting entire classes of similarly situated individuals. Second, the court in *Wyatt* held explicitly that there was a constitutional right to treatment applicable to mentally retarded people in institutions. *Wyatt* was the first case in which a court promulgated objectively measurable and judicially enforceable standards by which the right to treatment principle could be practically implemented. Finally, although only posing the possibility, the court emphatically stated its willingness to undertake responsibility for raising funds for and directly managing the implementation of constitutionally minimum standards, should the State of Alabama fail to do so. There is no doubt that the *Wyatt* case was closely watched by administrators and legislatures in other states with respect to its potential ramifications for them.

Willowbrook: Alternatives to Institutionalization Willowbrook was the next arena in which courts played a significant role in effecting major changes in the care of people with developmental disabilities. Willowbrook has become synonymous with poor institutional care, but it also represents the initiation of the phenomenon that characterizes the recent era in the field: deinstitutionalization.

As with the *Wyatt* case, it is ironic that the Willowbrook suit had its beginnings in the layoffs of employees at the Willowbrook State School in the spring of 1971. The problems at Willowbrook were not unknown before the suit was brought. Overcrowding, understaffing, and neglect of patients had been frequently brought to public attention by parent-advocacy groups, by state legislators, and in annual budget requests by the agency responsible for its administration. The conditions at Willowbrook were given statewide and national attention when Senator Robert F. Kennedy visited the institution in 1965. However, public protests by parents and employees concerning the effects of the layoffs and freeze on hiring in the fall of 1971, a series of newspaper exposes on the conditions at Willowbrook, and a television network special brought national attention to this situation.

A federal survey team under the leadership of the National Institute of Mental Health was organized; the Governor's Developmental Disabilities Council conducted a review, and a large number of other local, state, and federal officials toured the facility and called for various local, state, and federal actions to ameliorate the deplorable conditions. Governor Nelson Rockefeller provided some relief to the institution by lifting the hiring freeze (Castellani, 1975).

In March, 1972, two class action suits were filed in the U.S. Federal District Court seeking for the plaintiffs, who represented the residents at Willowbrook, comprehensive relief from the deleterious conditions and a restructuring of the delivery of services. The primary plaintiff was the New York State Association for Retarded Children, Inc.

The plaintiffs' complaint against the State of New York was a comprehensive attack on the system of care for the residents at Willowbrook. The conditions at Willowbrook which the plaintiffs sought to correct were grouped under three major categories: overcrowding, lack of staff, and *failure to provide community alternatives to institutionalization* (emphases added) (*ARC v. Rockefeller*, 1972).

Although the *ARC v. Rockefeller* suit was significant in that it addressed the issue of alternatives to institutionalization, the main thrust of the suit was to improve conditions *within the institution*. Moreover, the specific court orders in *ARC v. Rockefeller* focused on enhanced staffing, medical services, the use of seclusion and restraint, and other protections and guarantees that would serve to achieve those objectives. Indeed, the court in *ARC v. Rockefeller* took a more cautious position than the court in *Wyatt*. Instead of reaffirming that court's finding of a "right to treatment," the court in *ARC v. Rockefeller* based its findings on a more passive "right to protection from harm" (*ARC v. Rockefeller*, 1973). The various orders in the case did have the effect of relieving overcrowding by transferring residents to other facilities, but it was not until the Willowbrook Consent Decree in 1975 that the issue of deinstitutionalization was fully addressed. Nonetheless, the *ARC vs. Rockefeller* case did represent a continuation of the important new policy initiatives set in the *Wyatt* decision, and although the basis it set for deinstitutionalization moved through different policy processes, it served as a bridge to the *Pennhurst* case, which did indeed represent the apotheosis of judicial policy-making in this area.

Halderman v. Pennhurst State School and Hospital: Deinstitutionalization   As in the *Wyatt* (1972) and *ARC v. Rockefeller* (1972) cases, the Pennhurst (1978) case sought improvements in the conditions at the institution when the case was initiated in 1974 (Bradley, 1985). This case, which progressed through the courts after Wyatt and *ARC v. Rockefeller*, began to embody both the more widely accepted notions that large institutions were, *ipso facto*, inappropriate places for the care of people with developmental disabilities and the experience of large-scale deinstitutionalization that was indeed taking place in certain states. The plaintiffs ultimately expanded the remedies sought to encompass full-scale deinstitution-alization.

The *Pennhurst* case does constitute a major landmark in the field in that it was the first case dealing with mentally retarded people within institutions to reach the United States Supreme Court. However, the decisions in the case were "narrow and extremely cautious" (Bradley, 1985, p. 86) and did not themselves require the large-scale deinstitutionalization that was initiated through consent decree.

PARC v. Commonwealth: Free and Appropriate Education The *Pennsylvania Association for Retarded Children v. Commonwealth of Pennsylvania case (PARC v. Commonwealth,* 1972) is a major landmark case that has had important ramifications in the area of education of handicapped children. The parents' association at Pennhurst State Institution in Pennsylvania brought suit to address physical abuse and other institutional problems at that facility. However, rather than pursuing the right to treatment arguments as in *Wyatt v. Stickney* (1972) and *ARC v. Rockefeller* (1972), PARC pursued its objectives by attacking the school exclusion suffered by those individuals institutionalized at Pennhurst. The consent decree that resolved this initial suit established the principle that a state could not deny any mentally retarded child a free public education (Laski, 1985). The *PARC v. Commonwealth* case not only was one important base for the *Halderman v. Pennhurst* (1978) case that followed but it also laid a judicial foundation for the right to a free appropriate public education that was later embodied in the Education for All Handicapped Children Act (PL 94-142). Laski points out that *PARC* and the subsequent *Mills* case (*Mills v. D. C. Board of Education,* 1972) provided the foundation supporting the four major principles of the right to education: zero reject education, integrated education, appropriate education, and due process (Laski, 1985).

Consent Decrees Large-scale deinstitutionalization undertaken within the framework of judicial policy-making has come largely through the vehicle of consent decrees. Indeed, Bradley (1985) has suggested that in many states consent decrees have provided a convenient vehicle for sympathetic state administrators to effect, under the implied threat of judicial sanctions, systemic changes and deinstitutionalization that might not have otherwise occurred. In New York, Congressman Hugh Carey promised in his campaign for Governor to settle the *ARC v. Rockefeller* (1972) suit, and he signed the Willowbrook Consent Agreement in 1975. That set into motion a process of implementation to close Willowbrook. As the Rothmans describe in their book, *The Willowbrook Wars* (1984), the consent decree did not eliminate the adversarial relationship between the state and the plaintiffs (acting through the Willowbrook Review Panel), nor did it make the process of deinstitutionalization easy or free of substantial clashes of political will. It was nonetheless a process of implementation, albeit contentious, toward generally agreed-upon objectives.

Summary Two questions need to be addressed: What has been the impact of these judicial decisions, and most importantly, what effect will they have on the future of community-based developmental services? First, these decisions, consent decrees, and other actions taken within the framework of the judicial system cannot be considered in isolation. Other important policy initiatives were occurring at about the same time, and there were important reciprocal effects. These other developments are discussed in the next section, and their collective impact is considered at the end of this chapter. Nonetheless, the use of courts as vehicles to effect changes in the care of people with developmental disabilities has been an extremely important element in the field, and there are identifiable outcomes from those efforts.

In the first instance, the decision to seek redress through lawsuits forced advocates for people with developmental disabilities to be advocates in the true sense of the term. It would be unfair to characterize the organizations concerned with the care of people with developmental disabilities as lacking in aggressiveness before the era of judicial policy-making or to fault them for not having then the negative view of large institutions that prevails today. Whatever their previous stance, judicial policy-making is fundamentally adversarial (e.g., *Wyatt versus Stickney*, 1972). Parent advocacy organizations across the country directly challenged the administrations of operating institutions and the legislatures that appropriated funds for the care of their children. A heightened sense of advocacy for the rights of people with developmental disabilities was demonstrated in a number of ways at that time, but no policy process focuses that advocacy role as keenly as litigation. It might not be too speculative to suggest that the adversarial stance required in judicial processes served to enhance the aggressiveness of advocates in other policy arenas.

Judicial policy processes are substantially more specific and structured than typical administrative or legislative policy processes. In contrast to the relatively general advocacy for additional funds or new programs that characterizes these other policy processes, the progress of the various suits toward orders and decisions required the parties to the suit, and the judges themselves, to begin to define the remedies in very specific terms. Beginning with *Wyatt v. Stickney* (1972), these remedies took the form of specific actions or conditions that were: 1) explicit and measurable and 2) required to be achieved within definite time frames. Even though some of the early orders in *Wyatt v. Stickney* and *ARC v. Rockefeller* (1972) were only based on standards that were judicially mandated for prisoners (Castellani, 1975), the specificity of the stipulated outcomes and the timetables established for their attainment represented substantial departures in policy-making for people with developmental disabilities. Indeed, as the cases in this area developed, plaintiffs were forced to identify more carefully the specific remedies they sought, and it was largely through the progress of the several cases that those remedies became more progressive and eventually included the demand for abolition of large institutions.

A number of legislative and administrative actions occurred at the federal level during the 1970s that have had important ramifications for state and local governments. Nonetheless, the direct, immediate, and powerful involvement of federal courts in an area that had been the virtually exclusive province of state and local government policy had an enormous effect. Although judicial activism eventually affected a number of areas (school desegregation, for example), Judge Johnson's order in *Wyatt v. Stickney* (1972)—proferring a special master, calling for a special session of the state legislature to appropriate funds, and threatening seizure and sale of state lands to ensure those funds for court operation of the facility if necessary—sent a powerful message to state administrations and legislatures across the country. Although most deinstitutionalization efforts have taken place within the framework of consent decrees, it would be difficult to imagine states undertaking actions as broad as they have without the ultimate threat contained in Judge Johnson's order in 1972. Clearly, the redefinition of the policy problem as an abridgement of federal constitutional rights and guarantees triggered a new and powerful dimension of intergovernmental relations.

In general, it seems clear that courts have played an extremely important role in deinstitutionalization. They served to establish the decision-making framework of the process directly and indirectly, provided the vehicle for and the arbiter of the specific remedies and conditions sought for people with developmental disabilities, and galvanized the advocates for those individuals to take aggressive (and adversarial) actions on their behalf. How these actions related to other developments occurring in the field toward similar goals of deinstitutionalization is examined next, followed by a consideration of the effect of judicial policy-making on the creation of community-based services.

Legislation and the Creation of Community-Based Services

The judicial initiatives that were affecting institutions and community-based services during the early and mid-1970s were closely entwined with several legislative developments that made important contributions to the legal framework in this area. These included legislation affecting the education of handicapped children, the federal developmental disabilities legislation, vocational rehabilitation and related statutes, and changes in the financing of developmental services through Titles XIX and XX of the Social Security Act and through Supplemental Security Income.

The Education for All Handicapped Children Act (PL 94-142) The Education for All Handicapped Children Act of 1975 (PL 94-142) clearly stands out as one of the most significant elements of the legal framework of community-based services. The federal government had for a number of years provided aid to local school districts for services to educationally disadvantaged children (Braddock, 1987). The Elementary and Secondary Education Act Amendments of 1970 consolidated several separate special education statutes into a separate title referred to as the "Education of the Handicapped Act" (Braddock, 1987). In 1974 amendments to the statute (PL 93-380) required states to establish goals and plans for providing full educational opportunities for all handicapped children (Braddock, 1987).

The *PARC* and *Mills* cases were having a significant effect on the right to education issue in the mid-1970s, and Laski (1985) argues that Congress saw that the provision of educational services to handicapped children would prevent their institutionalization. The landmark 1975 legislation stipulates:

> A free appropriate public education will be available for all handicapped children between the ages of three and eighteen within the State not later than September 1, 1978 and for all handicapped children between the ages of three and twenty-one within the State no later than September 1, 1980. (Public Law 94-142, 1975, Section 612 (2) (B))

Although other sections of the statute served to exempt the states from full implementation in some respects, the standard—"a free appropriate public education"—has become a central principle in the legal framework of community-based services.

The enactment of PL 94-142 also expanded the State Grant Program in special education that began in 1967 to provide full educational opportunities for handicapped children. The State Grant Program directs that local and intermediate schools provide specially designed instruction to handicapped pupils based on *an individualized education program* (IEP). *Related services*, including transportation, developmental, corrective, or other supportive services to help the pupil benefit from the special education, are also required, and *due process guarantees* are also provided for in the legislation. These three elements form the basic structure of education for handicapped children.

Although those structural elements have had an important effect in improving educational opportunities, funding for special education remains problematic. As Braddock has pointed out, although the amount of federal funds made available through the State Grant Program has grown from $47.5 million in 1975 to over $1.1 billion in 1985, the program has not approached the 40 percent of the national average per pupil expenditure anticipated in the 1975 statute (Braddock, 1987). Indeed, he points out that funding for that program as of 1984 only represented approximately 10 percent of per pupil costs nationwide (Braddock, 1987).

Developmental Disabilities and Rehabilitation Legislation A number of federal statutes enacted during the 1970s were significant components of the legal framework that affected institutional and adult habilitation services. The Developmental Disabilities Services and Facilities Construction Act of 1970 was an important piece of federal legislation both in terms of its move toward service provision and in its embodiment of basic definitions in the field. As Braddock (1987) has pointed out in his extensive analysis of legislation in the area, the 1970 statute grew out of the Mental Retardation Facilities Construction Act of 1963, but replaced funds for construction with state formula grants that targeted planning and gap-filling services. The legislation also continued funding for the University Affiliated Facilities authorized in the 1963 legislation. These are research and training programs in developmental disabilities at major medical schools throughout the country.

The 1970 Developmental Disabilities Act was also a landmark in substituting the term "*developmental disability*" for "*mental retardation*." Cerebral palsy and epilepsy were identified as two additional developmental disabilities to be targeted for services under the act.

In 1973, the Rehabilitation Act (PL 93-112) revised and expanded the vocational rehabilitation program. Section 504 of that statute has become one of the major landmarks in the legal framework of deinstitutionalization and community-based services. Based in large measure on the language and approach of the Civil Rights Act of 1964, Section 504 prohibited exclusion from participation by an otherwise qualified handicapped individual in any program receiving federal funds (Braddock, 1987; Laski, 1985).

In 1975, the Developmental Disabilities Assistance and Bill of Rights Act amended the 1970 legislation in several important ways. First, states were required to spend at least 30 percent of their formula grants on deinstitutionalization activities and to incorporate deinstitutionalization into the state plans required by the statute. Second, the act contained a bill of rights for developmentally disabled people. Third, autism was included as a developmental disability.

The Rehabilitation, Comprehensive Services and Developmental Disabilities Amendments of 1978 (PL 95-602) extended the 1975 act and contained some important revisions. The 1978 statute changed the definition of developmental disability from the previously defined categories (mental retardation, cerebral palsy, epilepsy, autism and dyslexia) to a functional definition. According to the 1978 definition, developmental disability requires the presence of three or more substantial functional limitations among the seven major life activity areas: self-care, receptive and expressive language, learning, mobility, self-direction, capacity for independent living, and economic self-sufficiency. The 1978 legislation also authorized the establishment of protection and advocacy systems in the states. Finally, it called for a shift in services from planning to "priority services," which included case management, child development, alternative community living, and nonvocational social-developmental services.

The 1978 legislation was significant in also providing the basis for a distinct service model. It established grant authority for Independent Living Services for persons with severe disabilities. The 1978 amendments also modified greatly the service priorities of state vocational rehabilitation facilities by requiring them to give priority to clients with severe mental and physical handicaps.

The Developmental Disabilities Act of 1984 (PL 98-527) emphasized services necessary for people with developmental disabilities to achieve their maximum potential through increased independence, productivity, and integration into the community. Consistent with this focus, priority services were redefined to include employment-related activities, and nonvocational social-developmental services were deleted from that category.

Other Federal Legislation There were a wide variety of other federal statutes passed in the 1970s that affected deinstitutionalization and establishment of community-based services, although not with as far-reaching an impact as those described above.

Several pieces of federal legislation, such as the Maternal and Child Health State Formula Grant Program and the Crippled Children's Services State Grant Program (now Maternal and Child Health Block Grant), provided services of particular importance to prevention and early intervention in developmental disabilities (Braddock, 1987). A variety of research and training programs directly in and affecting the field of developmental disabilities received substantial increases in funding through the 1970s (Braddock, 1987). Small Business Act Handicapped Assistance loans to sheltered workshops and Housing and Urban Development (Section 202 and Section 8) loans for apartments and group homes were particularly important in establishing an array of community-based services for people with developmental disabilities. These and related federal statutes have become important components of the overall legal framework of the field.

State Legislation and Community-Based Services Hanley-Maxwell and Heal's (1980) review of state legislation affecting community integration of people with developmental disabilities emphasizes general enabling statutes and licensing regulations for group homes. Bates' recent survey of state zoning legislation affecting community residences is also an important review (1985). Although there are similar statutes in other states that have facilitated the development of group homes, a brief review of the New York State law, Section 41.34 of the Mental Hygiene Law, illustrates the important impact that state legislation has had on one crucial element of deinstitutionalization and the establishment of community-based services.

Section 41.34 of the Mental Hygiene Law, site selection of community residential facilities, is commonly referred to as the Padavan Law after the state senator who sponsored the legislation. This statute creates a notice, hearing, and appeal process for the establishment of community residential facilities for persons with disabilities. It allows a municipality to approve, suggest alternate sites, or object to selected sites. However, the final decision rests with the state commissioner, and although establishing a process with such standards as the concentration of such facilities, the law effectively removes from municipalities the capacity to block establishment of community residences. In light of the early widespread objections to community residences in many locales, this and similar statutes in other states have been an important element in the legal framework contributing to deinstitutionalization and the establishment of community-based services.

Summary Important programs mandated by the developmental disabilities and vocational rehabilitation acts include: university affiliated facilities, protection and advocacy systems, developmental disabilities planning councils, and independent living centers. These statutes have also codified the definition of developmental disability and identified the groups of individuals covered within it. The 1978 Rehabilitation Act amendments established service priorities among those individuals with different levels of disabilities.

The Education for All Handicapped Children Act, and subsequent amendments, is the primary vehicle defining, mandating, and guiding the provision of educational and related services to handicapped children. Although full implementation has been problematic, this legislation is clearly the cornerstone of this fundamental component of community-based services.

In summary, federal legislation during the 1970s played an important role in defining the parameters of the field of developmental disabilities by identifying its clientele and specifying its services. The legislation was particularly important in the field of education of handicapped children in acting as the basic charter, the source of federal funds (albeit insufficient), and, most important, the lever mandating the expenditure of state and local funds in this area. The legislation in the area of education, and in the others to a lesser extent, served to consolidate and codify the gains that advocates had made in various courts. As discussed below, the major sources of funds for deinstitutionalization and the establishment of community-based services came through legislation in related areas, but legislation in the developmental disabilities-vocational rehabilitation and special education areas was very important to establishing the legal framework in the area.

FINANCING DEINSTITUTIONALIZATION
AND COMMUNITY-BASED SERVICES

The financing of deinstitutionalization and community-based services has received a substantial amount of attention, and the role of public funding of community-based services is discussed in more detail in later chapters. However, to understand how the recent history of this field affects the future of community-based services, it is important to appreciate the central role of changes in the financing of services for people with developmental disabilities.

This section reviews how large increases in the amount of public funds expended for developmental services and changes in the ways in which those funds were made available have become central factors affecting the number of community-based services and the ways that they are provided. A very brief description of the basic parameters of the three major funding programs is presented in the following section. Several of the sources used in this chapter, particularly Braddock (1987) and Gettings (1980), contain excellent detailed descriptions and analyses of various funding programs.

Changes in the Amounts of Public Funding

As Gettings (1980) has pointed out:

> Prior to the mid-1960s the federal government expended practically no federal funds on services to mentally retarded children and adults. At the time, the only publicly financed services were provided through large, state-operated institutions serving both mentally retarded children and adults, and widely scattered public school classes for "educable" and sometimes "trainable" youngsters. (p. 1)

Public, especially federal government, spending for health and human services grew exponentially during the 1970s, and the growth in spending on services for people with developmental disabilities was a part of that overall trend. Nonetheless, although those increases represented substantial increments in other health and human services areas, the increases for services for people with developmental disabilities was a radical change.

In a recent review, Braddock concluded that from 1962 through 1984 federal assistance programs for mental retardation and developmental disabilities grew from $118 million to $7.4 billion per year (1986). Braddock and his associates have estimated the total federal, state, and local expenditures for developmental services to be between $15.4 and $17.2 billion in fiscal year 1984 (Braddock, 1987). Although the shifts among federal, state, and local spending are important, as well as the distribution between institutional and community-based services (and are considered in a later chapter), it should be apparent that the sheer magnitude of the increase in the amount of spending has been enormous.

Sources of Funding for Developmental Services

In addition to the sheer magnitude of the increases in public funding of services for people with developmental disabilities, the most important aspect of the funding has been that "the preponderance of federal dollars currently expended on behalf of mentally retarded clients are funneled through income maintenance, medical, and public assistance programs" (Gettings, 1980, p. 4). At the same time that the basic definitions, target populations, and service models of the field of developmental disabilities were being honed to a greater degree of specificity in the areas of legislation discussed above, most federal and related state funding for people with developmental disabilities was being channeled through health and human services entitlement programs.

Income Maintenance The *Supplemental Security Income (SSI)* program was created by Congress in 1972 (PL 92-603) as Title XVI of the Social Security Act. Title XVI repealed existing public assistance programs for blind, elderly, and disabled individuals and established a base federal income support level for these groups.

Eligibility for SSI was limited to individuals who had become disabled before age 22 and were not capable of "substantial gainful employment." The 1972 legislation also made children who were disabled eligible for SSI benefits if their disability was comparable in severity to that of adults. In 1984, over 600,000 people with mental retardation received SSI benefits through federal assistance payments and SSI state supplementation (Braddock, 1987).

Supplemental Security Income is a benefit of particular importance to disabled individuals living alone, at home, or in community-based residences. Monthly payments are made to individuals and couples, with an average individual monthly payment of $257 in 1984 (Braddock, 1987). Eligible individuals living and receiving support and maintenance in the household of another, such as a parent, receive one-third of the full SSI allowance. However, in some states individuals who live in state- or voluntary-operated community residences may qualify for a "congregate care" level of payment that is substantially greater than the amount paid to an individual living alone. An otherwise eligible person residing in a public institution or in a health care facility and receiving payments under Medicaid is limited to a $25 per month personal needs allowance. States have the option of supplementing federal SSI benefits, and 45 states and the District of Columbia do so. SSI benefit payments are tied to an individual's earnings and state vocational rehabilitation services. The incentives and disincentives of those linkages are discussed in more detail in Chapter 3.

Social Security Disability Insurance for Adult Disabled Children (SSDI) is the other major income maintenance program of importance to people with developmental disabilities. This program, which was originally authorized in 1956, provides for disability insurance payments to surviving disabled children age 18 or older of retired, deceased, or disabled workers who are eligible to receive Social Security benefits (Braddock, 1987). Disability is defined as an "inability to engage in any substantial gainful activity by reason of any medically determinable physical or mental impairment which can be expected to last for a continuous period of not less than 12 months."

Braddock (1987) estimates that the average monthly benefit payment in 1984 for an adult disabled child was $270. This figure is based on a total enrollment in 1984 of 503,000 recipients who were mentally retarded. That enrollment figure is exponentially greater than the 20,000 eligible beneficaries for the entire program estimated at the program's inception in 1956 and, according to Boggs (1981) shows the extent of disability due to mental retardation in the adult noninstitutionalized population.

In general, the SSI and SSDI income maintenance programs are enormous sources of funding both directly to disabled individuals and through them to community-based services. Braddock states that "federal income maintenance spending was the principal fiscal component of the federal mission in mental retardation for the 27-year period of FY 1950–76" (1987, p. 133). Braddock projects total income maintenance payments of over $3 billion in 1985 (1987).

Medical Assistance

Medicaid—Title XIX   The largest source of funding for services to people with developmental disabilities is the medical assistance program Medicaid—Title XIX of the Social Security Act—that was established in 1965. When created, it was regarded as a substantially less important part of the legislative effort that resulted in the Medicare program, and indeed, it differs from Medicare in several basic respects (Marmor, 1970).

The Medicaid program is a state-federal medical assistance program for the needy: those individuals who meet a means test and are categorically needy and those above the poverty level but who are designated as medically needy. The Medicaid program requires that states choose to participate and provide services according to a state plan, which must be approved by the Department of Health and Human Services, and which specifies the services that will be provided, including mandatory and optional services, and the criteria for eligibility in the program. The federal government reimburses states for 50–70 percent of the total *approved costs* of *approved services* to *eligible clients* delivered by *certified providers*.

In 1971 Congress passed legislation (PL 92-223) that transferred the intermediate care facility (ICF) program to Title XIX. Intermediate care services were to be delivered to individuals who did not need the intensive care of either a hospital or a skilled nursing facility, and the statute authorized the reimbursement of these services to mentally retarded and developmentally disabled individuals in public institutions as long as the services met the criterion of being "active treatment."

Clauser (1985) points out that through these acts Congress intended both to help states cover the rapidly increasing costs of institutional care and to prod the states to develop standards of quality care in the institutions that had come under increasingly negative scrutiny. The overall impact has been to increase enormously the federal share of funding institutional services. As Braddock notes, "ICF/MR funding is the single largest federal assistance program in mental retardation and developmental disabilities" (1987). More importantly, the Medicaid ICF/MR program resulted in a shift of fiscal responsibility from the states to the federal government for the operation of state facilities for people with developmental disabilities. As Braddock, Hemp, and Howes point out, "Between 1977 and 1984, the federal ICF/MR share of total nationwide expenditures for institutional services has doubled, growing from 23% to 45%" (1986, pp. 13–14). Overall, the federal ICF/MR program amounted to $2.66 billion dollars in 1985 (Braddock, 1987). Figure 2.1 shows the proportions and categories of federal, state and local MR/DD expenditures.

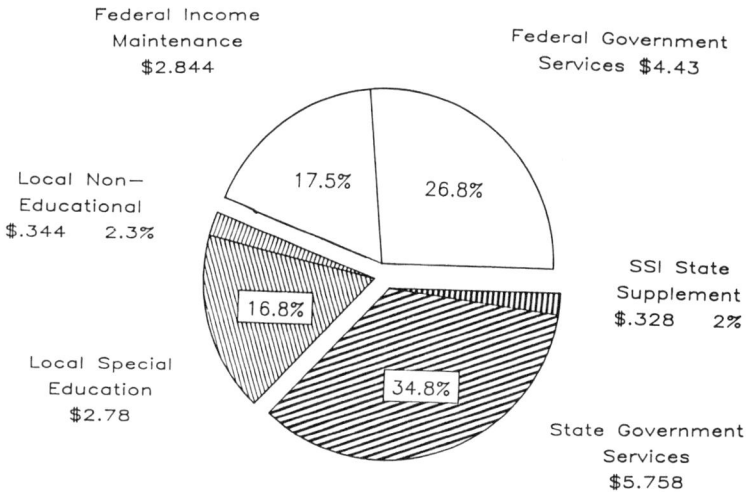

Federal Income
Maintenance
$2.844

Federal Government
Services $4.43

Local Non—
Educational
$.344   2.3%

17.5%   26.8%

16.8%

SSI State
Supplement
$.328   2%

Local Special
Education
$2.78

34.8%

State Government
Services
$5.758

Total MR/DD Expenditures: $16.488 Billion

Figure 2.1. Federal, state, and local spending for mental retardation and developmental disabilities in fiscal 1984, in billions of dollars. (Reprinted with permission from Braddock & Hemp, 1986, p. 706.)

CONCLUSION

This chapter has reviewed the important events and dimensions in the field of developmental disabilities in the past 10–15 years. Even this general review should make it clear that the forces and factors that have brought the field to this point in the evolution of community-based services for people with developmental disabilities continue to exert powerful political and programmatic energy. However, it seems that the impact of some of those forces may have become more diffuse. Also, the anomalies within and among the major policy dimensions may be more apparent and troublesome in the community context.

Political Ideology

There are several important conclusions with respect to political ideology. First, advocates for reform in the care of people with developmental disabilities have been guided by rather explicit political ideologies and continue to look to those concepts for clear guidelines for advocacy and standards against which to judge the adequacy of public policy. Second, there has been a shift over time in that political ideology from an initial focus on the civil rights of institutionalized clients to the concepts of normalization and the least restrictive alternative, which have underpinned deinstitutionalization. Nonetheless, the residual impact of that earlier paradigm can still be seen in direct advocacy by some parents (and policy-makers) to upgrade institutional care, as well as in the large and more pervasive effects of the application of large amounts of federal funds through the ICF/MR program to maintain large institutions. Although normalization and the abolition of institutions have become the more prevailing elements of the political ideology, the residual effects of those earlier concepts are substantial.

It remains to be seen to what extent normalization will continue to act as an important political ideology that provides relatively clear, salient guidelines for advocacy and policy-making in a community context. Normalization acted as a powerful political tool when the alternatives between institutional and community care were large and stark and will likely continue to do so in those situations. However, in the more complex environment of the community, the political and economic choices about which clients to serve and what services to deliver will be more subtle. This concept's most noted exponent, Wolf Wolfensberger, called into question the appropriateness of its use by many in the field (Wolfensberger, 1983). However, in light of the almost universal use of the term and acknowledgment of its importance, it is unlikely that even Wolf-ensberger's proposed reconceptualization will serve to change its current usage or establish a similarly important new line of thought. Yet, it is unlikely that the advocacy and political decision-making affecting the evolution of community-based services for people with developmental disabilities will be directed and measured against a cohesive and widely shared political ideology, such as normaliza-tion. Whether such notions as long-term care reform, services coor-dination and integration, or other such conceptual frameworks that seem to have some currency can act as powerfully to provide direc-tion to advocates and policy-makers in the community context also remains to be seen.

Legal Framework

Much of the judicial output in the 1970s was targeted to closing large institutions. Although the process of deinstitutionalization is not complete, the cautious and limited nature of recent decisions sug-gests that federal courts are unlikely either to take the lead or act as sympathetic agents in aggressively pursuing deinstitutionalization.

From a statutory perspective, it seems that the crucial problems lie in the area of implementation. During the 1970s federal legisla-tion was important in defining the basic parameters of the field in terms of clientele, services, and priorities. To a large degree, enhanc-ing the availability and accessibility of community-based services will depend on how well those parameters and elements can be applied at the local level. To some extent, adequate financing will be an important element and catalyst. However, it is also becoming clear that the separate development of major pieces of federal legisla-tion in developmental disabilities, vocational rehabilitation, and special education results in important anomalies and discontinuities in clientele, services, and priorities "at the point of delivery" in communities where their integration and coordination are crucial to the enhancement of community-based services.

Financing

A number of analysts have pointed out the major anomalies that exist in the financing of developmental services (Braddock & Hemp, 1986; Clauser, 1985; Fernald, 1986; Gettings, 1980). The most impor-tant sources of federal funding for community-based services are income maintenance and medical assistance programs. By far, Med-icaid funding of ICFs/MR has proven to be the most problematic. Although debates within the field over home and community care waivers and legislative proposals to defund large institutions have drawn substantial attention, the overarching concern is that the federal government is increasingly unsympathetic to health and human services programs in general and that deficit reduction measures will ultimately result in substantial diminution of federal funds to the entire field of developmental disabilities.

In many respects, establishment of community-based services has come about as the outcome of deinstitutionalization: they essentially provide services to the same clientele in different settings. As the following chapter points out, there is a strong possibility that community-based services will be called upon to serve new and larger numbers of people with developmental disabilities. However, there is no corresponding likelihood that more funds will be available to do so.

Thus, recent history seems to provide a mixed and uncertain set of guidelines for the future of community-based services. The field of developmental disabilities has undergone revolutionary change within the past 15 years. A redefinition of the field, the emergence of a powerful philosophy, extraordinary court decisions, major federal legislation, large-scale deinstitutionalization, important new programs in schools, and exponential increases in funding each carry with them an enormous political energy. The force and direction of each of these factors continue to have an important impact on the amounts of services and the ways which they are provided.

Important anomalies, however, are also involved in each of these phenomena. Moreover, their collective effect is somewhat uncertain as the problems of integrating and coordinating the various programs, clienteles, funding streams, and policy processes at the community level are still being addressed.

In the next four chapters, the major dimensions affecting the availability and accessibility of community-based services are explored. In each chapter, the impact of these forces from the recent history in the field is examined and assessed in the new community context and in relation to the new factors that have emerged in this environment.

3

The Economics
of Community-Based
Developmental Services

A BASIC PREMISE OF THIS BOOK IS THAT POLITICAL AND ECONOMIC FAC-
tors are inextricably entwined in affecting the availability and accessibility of services for people with developmental disabilities.
Another important premise is that a number of predominantly economic factors that affect the availability and accessibility of community-based services have remained largely unaddressed. These also
require examination and need to be integrated into a broader framework of analysis.

Conley's seminal work, *The Economics of Mental Retardation*
(1973), established a significant baseline for consideration of the
important economic issues in this area. A number of other subsequent analyses, particularly in the vocational field but also in other
areas, have focused on economic factors and have employed such
basic economic approaches as benefit-cost analysis (Boggs, 1981;
Bradley, 1981; Conley, 1985; Conley & Noble, 1985; Noble, 1985;
Thornton, 1985). These analyses are reviewed because of their central importance and relationship to other factors and dimensions and
because recent proposals for reform in financing are particularly
important to community-based services. There is, of course, a large
and growing body of literature on the public financing of developmental services. Because public funding does play such an important role in this area, the sources, amounts, and types of funding are
reviewed from the perspective of how they affect the availability and
accessibility of community-based services.

In addition to those issues of public finance, several other economic issues and factors have emerged that do not seem to have been
given sufficient attention within a framework that allows the consid-

eration of their interdependence and collective impact in the context of community-based services. As was pointed out in Chapter 1, a political economy perspective takes into account the impact of the environment of political and economic activity and provides a careful identification of the key actors whose behavior affects the outcomes that are our focus: the availability and accessibility of community-based services. This chapter examines the impact of the socioeconomic environment on the availability and accessibility of community-based developmental services, the reciprocal effects of the economic behavior of the disabled individual and various mechanisms of public funding and social insurance, and how the situation and behavior of the family of the disabled person affects access to services. Of particular importance is the role that the economics of provider organizations play in the availability and accessibility of services. The impact of such other key actors as employees is also outlined. Thus, the economic actions and impact on the individual, the family, the service organization, the service employee, and the socioeconomic environment should be seen as increasingly independent and interdependent factors in a political economy framework. An analysis of their individual and collective impact on the availability and accessibility of community-based developmental services can begin to address such fundamental concerns as the balance between public and private responsibility for the costs of developmental disabilities and the impact of market and public mechanisms on equity and efficiency.

PUBLIC FUNDING
OF COMMUNITY-BASED
DEVELOPMENTAL SERVICES

In the following sections such largely private factors as the impact of the community environment, the behavior of disabled individuals, the role of the family, and the economics of service organizations are discussed and their place in a comprehensive political economy perspective assessed. Nonetheless, the public financing of developmental services is clearly the most significant factor affecting their availability and accessibility because federal, state, and local government funding streams establish the basic context within which other public and private forces operate.

Several works have examined the financing of developmental services and the effects of proposals for reforms in the basic funding mechanisms and formulas (Boggs, 1979; Braddock, 1987; Fernald, 1986; Gardner, 1986; Gettings, 1980; Lakin, Hill, & Bruininks, 1985).

Braddock and his associates have devoted an exceptional amount of effort to analyzing the financing of developmental services, and their work constitutes an important comprehensive resource in this area (Braddock, 1987). Although this chapter briefly reviews the major sources and mechanisms of the public funding of developmental services, its primary concern is to explain how they affect the availability and accessibility of community-based developmental services. In addition, the chapter discusses how proposals for reform in the financing of developmental services and in the broader field of long-term care are likely to affect community-based services.

Medicaid and Developmental Services

In Chapter 2, several sources of funding of developmental services are described. Title XIX (Medicaid) has become the major fiscal force affecting the amount and structure of developmental services. Since 1971, Medicaid, largely through the Intermediate Care Facility/Mental Retardation (ICF/MR) program, has provided an exponential increase in federal funding of developmental services. More importantly, the CF/MR program has had the effect of underwriting the costs of institutional models of developmental services.

The ICF/MR program was initiated in the Social Security Amendments of 1971 (PL 92-223). Intermediate care facilities did not require the level of treatment typical of a hospital or skilled nursing facility, but involved "active treatment" in an institutional setting (Braddock, 1987). As Boggs points out, the transfer of the ICF program to Medicaid clearly required health-related care, and ICF residents were regarded as being in a "medical institution" (1981, p. 61). Nonetheless, the ICF/MR program allowed reimbursement for either medical care or habilitative care, in contrast to other Medicaid facilities in which only health-related care was reimbursed. The purpose of the "active treatment" requirement was to ensure that these funds were not used to support the custodial care in institutions, as was prevalent before the initiation of the ICF/MR program.

Of enormous importance was the authorization for public institutions to receive Medicaid reimbursement for the care and treatment of their residents. That is, the ICF/MR program provided the vehicle for states to recoup 50–78 percent of the costs of operating public institutions. Boggs, Lakin, and Clauser (1985) provide an excellent review of the background to this decision and point out that it had far-reaching consequences by directing substantial portions of federal funding through this program to institutions.

The ICF/MR program set into motion two important sets of forces that have significantly shaped the structure of developmental services. First, the regulations that were eventually promulgated in 1974 established standards for active treatment and particularly for physical plants that required states to upgrade their large public facilities in order to continue receiving Medicaid reimbursement under the program. Thus, the ICF/MR program requires states to invest funds in renovations and creates substantial incentives for the continued operation of newly refurbished (and bonded) institutions (Boggs, 1981; Boggs et al., 1985; Conley & Noble, 1985; Fernald, 1984; Gettings, 1980). Second, the ICF/MR program allows for community-based ICFs/MR so that states and other private provider organizations can also receive Medicaid reimbursement for smaller facilities more likely to be in community settings. Thus, the Medicaid-funded ICF/MR program has become the vehicle for states to shift a large proportion of their costs of operating public facilities for people with developmental disabilities to the federal government. As pointed out earlier, if Medicaid provided the vehicle, a variety of federal court decisions, orders and arrangements of consent decrees provided much of the stimulus. Boggs et al. (1985) describe the thinking of the National Association for Retarded Citizens leadership (of which Boggs was an important leader) in the early 1970s in advocating for the changes in the Social Security Act that would ensure federal funding of residential and developmental programming in both public and private facilities.

In the 1977 changes in the ICF/MR regulations, the Department of Health and Human Services required states to draw up plans of compliance that involved large reductions in the populations of the state institutions in order to continue to receive Medicaid reimbursement for those facilities. State governments soon found themselves involved in complex trade-offs set in motion by the fiscal dynamics of the ICF/MR program, SSI payments to people with developmental disabilities, plans of compliance, and consent decrees. Gettings (1980) provides a graphic example of how those fiscal dynamics affected the mix of options in Nebraska, which was one of the first states to undertake large-scale deinstitutionalization and which set a pattern that has been followed in a number of other states. As shown in Table 3.1, the placement of Beatrice State Developmental Center (BSDC) residents into Medicaid-reimbursable ICFs/MR in the community resulted in a substantial shift in the fiscal burden from the state to the federal government. Even the increased fiscal burden on counties still resulted in a major net reduction of overall state and local government expenditures, although the increased burden on county government is an issue that is discussed below.

Table 3.1. Fiscal impact of placement of clients at Beatrice State Developmental Center (692 clients at Placement Level 2, including 262 clients at Beatrice State Developmental Center and 430 clients in community placements)

Funding source	Existing funding formula	Title XIX funding formula	Impact increase (decrease)
State government	$11,239,200	$6,025,400	($5,213,800)
Federal government	5,937,500	9,779,300	3,841,800
County government	328,200	1,700,200	1,372,000
School districts	200,000	200,000	
Client payments	692,000	692,000	
Total funding required	$18.396,900	$18,396,900	

Source: Gettings (1980), p. 22; reprinted by permission.

It is important to understand that the options outlined above are made possible in large measure because the Medicaid-funded ICF/MR program is an open-ended entitlement program. The absence of clear-cut agreement on assessment of need or definition of active treatment made it possible to move a wide variety of clients into ICFs/MR and/or to convert existing noncertified facilities to ICFs by meeting staffing, programming, and physical plant standards largely without regard to whether the clients met some objectively measurable standard of need. It is also extremely important to appreciate the fact that Medicaid reimbursement is cost-based. That is, the federal government pays 50–78 percent of what states or other ICF providers spend to operate those facilities. The ability to include a wide range of individuals in the ICF/MR program, as well as the shift of a major portion of the cost of operating them to the federal government, created powerful incentives to employ this program as the preferred option in both community and institutional care for people with developmental disabilities. Indeed, as Braddock and his associates have described, the ICF/MR program has rapidly grown to become the largest source of federal funding for developmental services (Braddock, Hemp, & Howes, 1985b).

There have been a number of critiques of the adverse effects of the ICF/MR program on the availability and accessibility of community-based developmental services, particularly for individuals with developmental disabilities who have never been institutionalized (Boggs, 1981; Braddock & Hemp, 1986; Conley & Noble, 1985; Fernald, 1984, 1986; Gardner, 1986; Lakin, Hill, & Bruininks, 1985).

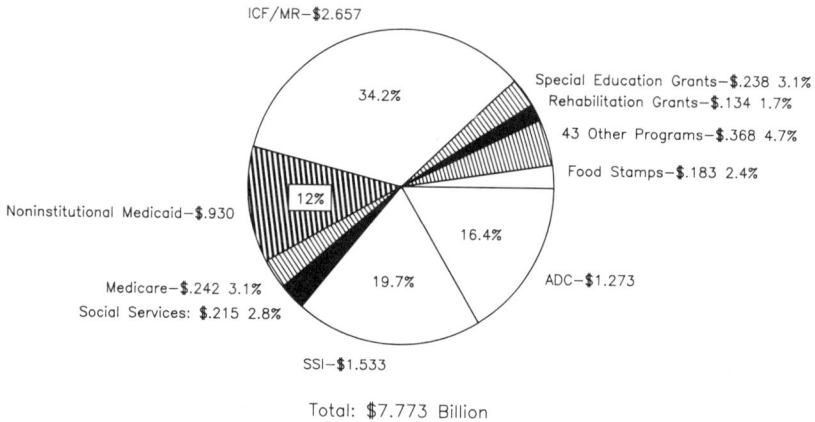

ICF/MR—$2.657

Special Education Grants—$.238 3.1%
Rehabilitation Grants—$.134 1.7%

43 Other Programs—$.368 4.7%

Food Stamps—$.183 2.4%

34.2%

12%

16.4%

Noninstitutional Medicaid—$.930

19.7%

ADC—$1.273

Medicare—$.242 3.1%
Social Services: $.215 2.8%

SSI—$1.533

Total: $7.773 Billion

Figure 3.1. Federal MR/DD spending by program in FY 1985 (dollars in billions). (Reprinted with permission from Braddock, D. [1987] *Federal Policy toward mental retardation and developmental disabilities* [p. 183]. Baltimore: Paul H. Brookes Publishing Co.)

First, the ICF/MR program is very expensive both as a program model and in the aggregate. It comprises 34 percent of total federal expenditures for developmental services; in comparison, only about 3 percent of federal government expenditures covers the costs of services to children with developmental disabilities in special education programs (Braddock, Hemp, & Howes, 1985b). That is, federal expenditures for ICF/MR care are 10 times greater than expenditures for special education. Figure 3.1 shows the relative proportions of federal funds by program. Although the escalation in ICF/MR costs is mirrored in the rise of overall expenditures for Medicaid, it is clear that the magnitude of these expenditures has brought a number of proposals for cost containment that will affect virtually all sources and mechanisms of funding for developmental services (Fernald, 1986; Gardner, 1986; National Study Group on State Medicaid Strategies, 1983). Because the funds from the ICF/MR program are overwhelmingly devoted to institutional costs, caps or stringent limits on funding growth overall tend to "lock in" the current institutional bias of federal funding. Moreover, the large absolute amounts and proportion of total federal expenditures in the ICF/MR program are devoted to a relatively small percentage of people with developmental disabilities (Braddock, Hemp, & Howes, 1985b).

Medicaid Waivers—Community and Family Living Amendments

The widespread concern both for the rapidly escalating costs of Medicaid and that the preponderance of federal funds was being devoted to institutional programs, rather than service models more fully integrated into the community, has led to two major responses in the field.

The Home and Community Care Waiver was passed as a part of the Omnibus Budget Reconciliation Act of 1981 (PL 97-35). The waiver allows the Department of Health and Human Services to permit states to finance community services through Medicaid for people who would otherwise be institutionalized in an ICF/MR. However, it requires that the average per capita cost of such services be lower than institutional care. Twenty-five states participated in the waiver, with the objectives of preventing admissions to ICFs/MR, facilitating deinstitutionalization, developing community-based alternatives to ICFs/MR, and integrating waived services into other community services (Gardner, 1986). Among the services in the various state proposals were respite care, special therapy services, parent training, and habilitation services in day and residential programs (Gardner, 1986).

Experience with the waivers has been rather problematic. There have been problems of implementation in several states, and some waivers merely shifted services funded under Title XX to Medicaid (Gardner, 1986). Moreover, the federal Health Care Finance Administration adopted a policy that effectively limited the number of Medicaid recipients so that states could not maximize the savings by serving more eligible clients and families. The waiver program, in general, does not allow for vocational and prevocational services that many professionals believe are vitally important community services, although the Consolidated Omnibus Budget Reconciliation Act of 1986 does make limited provision for funding vocational services under Medicaid. Finally, the waiver program is a time-limited program. There is evidence that states have become increasingly reluctant to rely heavily on the community-based approaches initiated under the waiver because they are uncertain about its long-term prospects as a source of funding for community-based developmental services (Gardner, 1986; NASMRPD, 1984).

A potentially more permanent change in federal funding for developmental services is the Community and Family Living Amendments of 1985 (S. 873) introduced by Senator John Chafee of Rhode Island. This proposed legislation would permanently restructure Medicaid services for people with developmental disabilities by authorizing Medicaid to pay for habilitative vocational and support services for people living at home or in small community living facilities; it would also establish strong fiscal disincentives to Medicaid reimbursement for services in large institutions. By broadening the range of Medicaid services, establishing criteria that would allow services to people not presently eligible, and creating fiscal incentives for states to develop additional community services, the Community and Family Living Amendments are expected to provide an important impetus to financing community-based developmental services. By requiring states to maintain their levels of expenditures while facing a gradual reduction of Medicaid reimbursement for ICFs/MR with more than 15 beds, the proposal intends to push states further away from institutional models of care.

In contrast to the relatively limited Home and Community Care Waiver program, the Community and Family Living Amendments would involve a more substantial change in the federal funding of developmental services through Medicaid. The proposal has attracted a wide base of support among advocacy groups, especially the Association for Retarded Citizens of the United States, and virtually all key actors seem to support its objectives. Nonetheless, several states with substantial numbers of clients in large ICF/MR facilities have viewed the proposal with some concern because of the investments they made to improve those institutions in order to qualify originally for reimbursement. A variety of changes have been made in the proposed bill to soften the penalties that those states would incur, and as in all legislative processes, it is likely that further compromises and adjustments will be negotiated. It seems that most advocates and professionals in the field of developmental disabilities are in favor of the basic thrust of the Community and Family Living Amendments so that some reform in that direction is likely to occur.

Federal Spending for Education, Social Services, and Income Maintenance

In contrast to the substantial increase in federal funding of institution-based services through the ICF/MR program, federal funding for education of children with handicaps has been substantially below expectations. Braddock points out that, although the original statute (PL 94-142) called for an escalating percentage of federal aid ultimately reaching 40 percent of the average per pupil expenditure, that commitment has not been realized. Moreover, the Omnibus Budget Reconciliation Act of 1981 changed that funding formula (Braddock, 1987). Federal spending for special education in 1985 amounted to approximately $1.135 billion (Braddock, 1987). Although the aggregate amount of federal, state, and local government funding of special education is difficult to calculate, it is nonetheless clear that the federal government's contribution to this central community-based service is not commensurate with the expectations of PL 94-142.

A relatively broad range of community-based social services had been available to people with developmental disabilities under Title XX of the Social Security Act. This program originally provided the greatest degree of integration among services for people with developmental disabilities in community settings. However, the generic nature of the funding made it difficult to identify specific service to that clientele, and it is likely that the lack of clear-cut linkages between services and clientele undercut its political support. As a result, in 1980, changes in the legislation (PL 96-272) established an expenditure ceiling, and in 1981 Title XX was converted into the Social Services Block Grant (Braddock, 1987), reducing federal reimbursements under this program in real economic terms until it accounted for only 7 percent of expenditures for community-based services by 1984 (Braddock, Hemp, & Howes, 1985c).

Income maintenance programs have been the major source of federal funding for developmentally disabled people living in community settings since 1950. The Supplemental Security Income (SSI) and Social Security Disability Insurance for Adult Disabled Children (SSDI) disbursed approximately $2.8 billion in 1985, and with food stamps, funded at $183 million in 1985, the total federal expenditure for income maintenance for persons with developmental disabilities was almost $3 billion (Braddock, 1987). Approximately one-fourth of all SSI recipients with disabilities in 1984 were people with mental retardation (Braddock, 1987). Although income maintenance is an especially important source of funding for non-ICF/MR community residential programs, the growth of federal income maintenance funding has leveled off, and there has actually been a decline in real economic terms in the past 2 years (Braddock, 1987).

State and Local Government Funding

Braddock, Hemp, and Howes (1985b) have pointed to the rapid and continuing growth of state funds in community-based services. Overall, state funds account for over 70 percent of total public spending on community-based services in 1984. However, their analysis of the changes in the patterns of public funding of community-based services also indicates that the relative commitment of state dollars vis-à-vis other sources has remained almost constant and indeed has actually declined by .1 percent between 1977 and 1984 (Braddock, Hemp, & Howes, 1985b).

The amount of local funding of community-based services is very difficult to estimate. A substantial portion of local public funding is devoted to the education of handicapped children under the mandates of PL 94-142. However, children with developmental disabilities are only one group of students with disabilities, and there have been long-standing problems in identifying that group and the costs associated with their education (Kakalik, Fury, Thomas, & Carney, 1981). Yet, there is no question that local governments, including school districts, have almost universally argued that they have had to bear a disproportionate share of the costs of special education. Braddock and Hemp calculate the costs of special education to localities to be approximately $1.27 billion, estimating that 10 percent of all handicapped children have mental retardation (1986).

Local governments also bear a portion of the cost of the ICF/MR program. In New York State, for example, the 50 percent total state contribution was actually comprised of a 25 percent local share and a 25 percent state share. Although the conversion of noncertified community residences to ICFs/MR and the use of that model for new residential programs resulted in an overall net transfer of the fiscal burden to the federal government, this program did make local governments (counties in New York State) fiscally liable for a portion of the costs of community-based services. In New York State the assumption of this and other Medicaid costs led to the passage of legislation that exempted localities from these Medicaid costs. However, localities have contributed substantial amounts of funds to other programs and services for people with developmental disabilities.

In addition to general social and health care services that localities provide to both disabled and nondisabled citizens, the cost of preschool services constitutes another increasingly large fiscal commitment for local governments. States vary in the distribution of responsibility between school districts and other local government agencies for funding and providing specific services to preschool children. In any case, the overall costs can be high, and as in New York State, these costs are borne by local governments to a considerable degree. In New York, a major portion of preschool services are directed through local (county-based) family courts, and the total statewide expenditures for preschool children with disabilities in 1985 was $180 million, of which the counties paid one-half the cost. As with school programs for children with disabilities, it is very difficult to estimate the proportion of clients, services, or costs specific to children with developmental disabilities. Local governments do nevertheless contribute an important amount of the financing of these services.

Summary

The major sources of public funding for developmental services—both institutional and community-based—are not dedicated exclusively to developmental disabilities. The most prominent example is the ICF/MR program, which is, at its core, a health-related institutional program. Virtually all the other important funding sources are not specific to developmental disabilities, which in one way or another confounds the availability and accessibility of a broad range of community-based services.

A second important feature of public funding of developmental services is the lack of programmatic or administrative coordination. There are major anomalies and discontinuities across public programs for people with developmental disabilities that make the implementation of comprehensive and coordinated services extremely problematic. For example, eligibility criteria for access to services change radically across the age spectrum so that the mandates of PL 94-142 (albeit poorly funded) are bracketed by similarly situated but underserved preschool and "aged out" people with developmental disabilities. The vagaries of Medicaid eligibility, as well as prior institutionalization, as factors affecting access, are dealt with in Chapter 4 and are symptomatic of the lack of coordination among major public programs in the area. The distribution of responsibility for funding, administration, and provision of services among various federal, state, and local government authorities is also an important feature of the uncoordinated nature of public programs.

Finally, as advocates, policy-makers, and service providers in all sectors turn increasingly toward the implementation of community-based developmental services, it appears that the public fiscal commitment to these services has plateaued. Despite the widely acknowledged problems inherent in Medicaid funding, for example, large increases in funding in this and other programs raised expectations that new community-based services would be financed from new funds. The Medicaid waiver program and the debate around the Community and Family Living Amendments proposal suggest that the further development of community-based programs may only come about through politically and administratively difficult trade-offs (and trade-ins) within existing funding levels.

THE SOCIOECONOMIC
ENVIRONMENT OF DEVELOPMENTAL SERVICES

Virtually since the inception of large-scale community-based programs for people with developmental disabilities, a number of analysts have pointed out the importance of such community-based services and resources as transportation, recreation, and medical services to the success of community living for these individuals (Bachrach, 1981; Gollay, Freedman, Wyngaarden, & Kurtz, 1978; Intagliata, Kraus, & Willer, 1980; Savage, Novak, & Heal, 1980). However, a careful reading of this literature indicates its relatively narrow focus with respect to the factors in the community that might affect the availability and accessibility of developmental services. Many examinations of the environment of community services focus on the architecture and design of housing, the number of individuals in programs, and management practices (Rotegard, Bruininks, Holman, & Lakin, 1985; Wolfensberger & Thomas, 1983). Other analyses point to inappropriate "values" and concern with the cost of services on the part of local legislators and school administrators as inhibiting implementation (Bruininks & Lakin, 1985). The organizational structure of local services (Gettings, 1981) and the level of urbanization (Minnesota Developmental Disabilities Program, 1983) are other factors that are noted in this context. However, there seems to be very little in the way of a systematic or comprehensive approach to the question of what factors or conditions in a community contribute to or inhibit the amount of services available or the ways in which they are delivered. Conversely, other than some concern with the effect of community residences on housing values (Wolpert, 1978), there is almost no attention paid to the reciprocal impact of community-based developmental services on the communities within which they are situated.

A review of literature and materials on the topic in general suggests that the shortcomings noted above are not unique to the field of developmental disabilities. Nonetheless, it seems that if the availability and accessibility of community-based services do indeed involve coordination and integration with existing community services and dependence on the values and resources of communities, then some attempt must be made to identify the factors in the community environment that are important and to consider how they might affect developmental services.

The definition of community is a complex and confounding issue throughout this and related discussions in later chapters. As is examined in greater detail in Chapter 6, we live in many geographic and functional "communities." From the perspective of the person with a developmental disability, his or her immediate neighborhood, school district, various local governments, and state all have important and distinct effects on the amount of developmental services available and that person's access to them.

General Economic Conditions

It would seem that both public and private expenditures for services for people with developmental disabilities would be related to the general ability of the government to pay for those services. However, a general review of the history of those expenditures in the past 10–15 years indicates that a curious political-economic dynamic is at work. During the 1970s when the national economy was generally sluggish and experiencing two recessions, public expenditures for developmental services increased dramatically (Braddock, 1986). Indeed, public expenditures for health during the 1970s were among the major contributors to the relatively high rates of inflation during that decade (HCFA Forum, 1981). Spivey (1985) has examined economic growth rates and expansion in welfare expenditures and found escalating expenditures in that area in an era of slow growth.

In contrast to the escalating expenditures for developmental services in the 1970s, as well as for health and welfare in general, public expenditures have plateaued in the past few years despite a generally improved national economy during that period (Braddock, 1986). Clearly, the policy choices that have been made by the Reagan Administration and the Congress (Omnibus Budget Reconciliation Act, Gramm-Rudman-Hollings, and other acts) suggest that the general health of the national economy is not a good predictor of the rate of public expenditures for developmental services. Indeed, although the history of large-scale community-based developmental services is relatively short, it seems that political rather than general economic factors have been most important in determining the rate of federal expenditures for developmental services.

State Economies and Developmental Services

The study of the relationships between levels of economic development and political attributes of national governments has been a concern of social scientists for some time (Lipset, 1959; Rostow, 1964). Studies of the relationships between the socioeconomic environments of state political systems and the policy outcomes in those states suggest one possible framework for addressing issues in the developmental disabilities field (Dawson & Robinson, 1963; Dye,

1966; Hofferbert, 1968, 1974; Sharkansky, 1967). In general, these studies have suggested that public policy outcomes in health and welfare are significantly related to such measures of the socioeconomic environment as levels of wealth, industrialization, urbanization, and education. Indeed, policy outcomes were generally found to be more significantly related to those socioeconomic factors than to the more traditional political process/structure factors, such as level of two-party competition. The approach used and conclusions reached by these analysts have been the source of considerable controversy (Hofferbert, 1974). Although the linkage among those socioeconomic variables, policy process and structure variables, and policy outcomes remains problematic, these analysts have served to sensitize social scientists to the important impact of the environment of the political system on policy processes.

Braddock and his associates completed an exhaustive descriptive statistical summary of state and national patterns of public funding of developmental services (Braddock, Hemp, & Howes, 1984). They ask, "To what extent, if any, do state variations in MR/DD fiscal performance relate to high levels of education or personal income among the general population" (Braddock et al., 1984, p. 86). They also suggest that funding be examined in relation to a variety of political factors as well. Because state expenditures are a large and crucial component of overall funding of community-based services, it is clear that these questions should be pursued to assess the impact on developmental services at the local level.

The Socioeconomic Context of the Community

The analyses above identify some of the factors that should have an important effect on the availability and accessibility of developmental services at the community level. Indeed, level of urbanization has been used as a locational factor in examining differences in per diem rates in community-based Intermediate Care Facilities across Minnesota (Minnesota, 1983; Wieck, 1980; Wieck & Bruininks, 1981). However, it is at the local community level that the impact of those factors is most directly felt and their effect most difficult to assess. Although aggregate measures of wealth, urbanization, education, and industrialization may typify states and affect levels of state expenditures, there are likely to be wide variations on those dimensions among locales within a state. Nonetheless, it should be possible to identify some important factors, begin to examine how they can be measured, and consider their effect on community-based services.

The basic dimensions outlined in the literature discussed earlier provide a framework with which to examine the impact of socioeconomic factors on the availability and accessibility of developmental services. Census data are readily available for areas small enough to measure general levels of local wealth, urbanization, industrialization, racial-ethnic composition, and education. In addition to measures of socioeconomic capacity, it should also be possible to begin to address the question of community values raised by Bruininks and Lakin (1985). By examining such indices as local tax levies compared to tax base expenditures per pupil from local tax levies and United Fund (Way) contributions per capita, measures of community willingness (an index of generosity?), as well as capacity to finance local services for people with developmental disabilities, can be developed (Bahl, 1984; Parker, 1985). Of course, measuring the impact of these factors on the availability of developmental services presumes that measures of the capacity of developmental services can be established. This is possible for many core residential and day services (beds, sheltered workshop capacity, etc.). It becomes very difficult as less routine and structured services, such as family supports, become available and people with developmental disabilities use such generic community services as transportation and recreation. The complexity of this approach should not be underestimated.

In addition to these general measures of capacity and willingness, there are several other important factors in the socioeconomic environment of services that must be identified, even if their place in an analytic scheme is difficult to determine. Housing costs, for example, are a major factor affecting the establishment of community residences. There are often wide variations in the cost of housing among locales, and the cost in some urban areas is so high as to be almost prohibitively expensive for the establishment of any substantial number of residences for people with developmental disabilities. The availability of housing (vacancy rates) and the compatibility of housing (multiple-story apartments) in urban areas for group homes for people with physical disabilities are important factors affecting the availability and accessibility of these residential services.

The cost and availability of labor are other important factors that must be taken into account. Although higher wage and salary rates in urban areas may be accounted for in cost-based reimbursement, this level of reimbursement is not likely to continue as an automatic escalator with the current move toward caps and block grant-type funding. High labor costs in a locale might have a negative effect on the ability of an agency to establish developmental services, although high labor costs are usually found in wealthier communities that can support more services. The availability of human service employees in general and specialized professionals, such as physical therapists, speech therapists, and occupational therapists, varies considerably, and greater numbers of specialized professionals are typically found in high-wage communities. In either case, availability of these individuals in communities has an important impact on the availability and accessibility of services.

The local labor market also has an important impact on the ability of people with developmental disabilities to secure employment, whether it be competitive, supported, or sheltered. High rates of unemployment, prevailing wages, and opportunities for employment of people with developmental disabilities are important aspects of the labor market and components of the socioeconomic environment of a community.

Other elements of the local environment that are important to people with developmental disabilities include the availability of transportation and the distance or ease of travel to services. Recreational resources and opportunities are also important, as well as the availability of general health, medical, and dental services. Census data on hospital beds and physicians per 10,000 people provide some rough indicators of human service capacity in a locale, but overall it is extremely difficult to measure these variables and even more difficult to assess their impact on services for people with developmental disabilities.

Impact of Developmental Services on the Community

As pointed out in Chapter 1, one benefit of a political economy perspective is that economics provides for an assessment of income, as well as expenditures. Or as put in one succinct analysis of potential cuts in public funding: "Remember, every dollar of expenditure is someone's dollar of income." When considering the socioeconomic environment within which developmental services are situated, it is also important that one takes into account the reciprocal economic impact of these services on the community.

Analyses of the effect of community residences on property values (Dolan & Wolpert, 1982; Ryan & Coyne, 1985; Wolpert, 1978) is one step in this direction, but that has not been generally pursued with related studies. The potential and actual closures of large institutions have again brought the economic issue to the fore as the loss of jobs, the cancellation of contracts for supplies, and other results of closure pose the prospect of substantial economic impact on the communities in which those institutions are located (Braddock & Heller, 1985; Conroy & Bradley, 1985; Minnesota State Planning Agency, 1985).

Yet, there seems to have been virtually no systematic attention to the positive economic effects on communities of the establishment of community-based services even though community-based services represent a growing element of the human service sector at the local level. In some rural communities sheltered workshops are among the largest employers both in terms of human service workers and persons with developmental disabilities (New York State ARC, 1985). One county mental health (including MR/DD) director in New York undertook a detailed analysis of community-based services and reported to the county legislature that those services "brought about a financial benefit to the County by bringing in additional State dollars and employment for local residents who now provide services" (Pepper, 1978, p. 45). He concluded that "the overall economic impact is positive because of the mental hygiene and human service industry that is created and supported by State and Federal dollars" (Pepper, 1978, p. 45). These data and analyses indicate that a more comprehensive and systematic examination of the economic impact of community-based developmental services might be important to enhancing their availability by showing their positive reciprocal effect on the community.

Summary

In general, there seem to be a number of possible approaches to identifying the factors in the socioeconomic environment of communities and assessing their impact on the availability and accessibility of developmental services. There are also many problems in identifying and assessing the impact of these factors. Nevertheless, it is crucial that, at the minimum, there be a greater sensitivity to the fact that the services and resources that are needed by people with developmental disabilities vary among locales and are to a large extent dependent upon and related to the socioeconomic environment. The ability to enhance those services and to adjust for the variation among and within communities requires a broadening of the analytic perspective to take into account routinely the socioeconomic environment.

PERSONS WITH DEVELOPMENTAL DISABILITIES
AND THE ECONOMICS OF DEVELOPMENTAL SERVICES

In a substantial amount of the literature in the field, people with developmental disabilities are discussed either implicitly or explicitly in ways that suggest their passive involvement in developmental services. The capacity of individuals with more severe disabilities to participate in choices of program and other important decisions about their lives is often limited. Nonetheless, the effect of the implementation of a broad range of community-based developmental services on these individuals' economic circumstances and their program preferences should be considered.

In this section two major issues are addressed. First, a substantial proportion of people with developmental disabilities *can* and *do* work. Their employment opportunities and their expectations, as well as those of employers and human service professionals, are crucial, and those choices affect their own access to services and ultimately the availability and accessibility of developmental services in communities. Second, this section examines the major sources of financial support for a developmentally disabled individual living in the community and assesses how the interplay among various funding sources creates economic dynamics that affect an individual's access to developmental services.

Employment Opportunities

Conley (1973) pointed out that a substantial proportion of adults with mental retardation living in the community were employed and were vocationally successful. He argued that several factors affected vocational success, including the demand for labor, the level and type of an individual's disability, place of residence, the attitude of the disabled person toward employment, and the attitude of employers toward hiring people with mental retardation. Conley also argued that an individual's level of intellectual deficiency, except in cases of severe retardation, was usually not the major factor in vocational success or failure (Conley, 1973). Since Conley's work a growing body of literature has consistently demonstrated the capacity of people with developmental disabilities to work in the competitive labor market (Kiernan, 1979; Kiernan & Ciborowski, 1985; Kiernan & Stark, 1986; Paine, Bellamy, & Wilcox, 1984; Wehman, 1981). These observations are consistent with those analysts in the broader field of disability, employment, and social insurance who have demonstrated that self-definition, work history, and other social and economic factors are more significant predictors of a person's capacity to obtain and hold a job than ostensibly objective physical criteria (Berkowitz, Johnson, & Murphy, 1976; Howards, Brehm, & Nagi, 1980; Rubin, 1978, 1982; Stone, 1984). Indeed, one of the findings of the recent major transitional employment demonstration—Structured Training and Employment Transitional Services (STETS)— was that the program was more successful for moderately retarded individuals than for those with borderline retardation (Kerachsky, Thornton, Bloomenthal, Maynard, & Stephens, 1985). The obvious conclusion from this growing body of literature is that employment, even in the competitive labor market, is within the capacity of a substantial number of people with developmental disabilities.

Despite the evidence that most people with developmental disabilities can work in the mainstream of the labor market, a large number of these individuals have been segregated from employment. In addition to being largely restricted from the free and appropriate education that would provide them with the needed skills for work, these people were largely excluded from traditional sheltered workshops until at least the 1950s. It was not until the 1970s that federal legislation began to have an important impact on the employment of people with developmental disabilities.

The Rehabilitation Act Amendments of 1973 (PL 93-112) provided for the expansion of vocational rehabilitation programs, and Section 504 of the statute prohibited discrimination in these and other programs against otherwise qualified individuals. The Education for All Handicapped Children Act of 1975 (PL 94-142) has also greatly expanded the vocational opportunities of people with developmental disabilities by enabling them to enter schools in greater numbers and to acquire a wide range of skills and experiences that are crucial to vocational success. The Rehabilitation Comprehensive Services Act and Developmental Disabilities Amendments of 1978 (PL 95-602) had a substantial effect on employment of disabled individuals by authorizing Independent Living Services, requiring Individual Written Rehabilitation Plans, and mandating state vocational rehabilitation agencies to give priority to clients with severe mental and physical handicaps. Both the 1973 and 1978 rehabilitation statutes authorized special demonstration projects that ultimately formed the basis of transitional and supported work programs (Braddock, 1987). Employment of people with developmental disabilities continued as a focus of federal legislation in the 1980s. The Developmental Disabilities Act of 1984 (PL 98-527) redefined priority services to include employment-related activities.

In addition to rehabilitation, education, and developmental disabilities statutes, several other pieces of federal legislation have had an important effect on enhancing the employment opportunities of people with developmental disabilities. The Comprehensive Employment and Training Act (CETA) provided many developmentally disabled people with jobs, and the Job Training Partnership Act (JTPA) has also targeted handicapped people for employment and training (Kerachsky et al., 1985). There is also, however, some evidence to suggest that the stigma attached to the disadvantaged worker covered by JTPA may harm that person's job prospects (Burtless, 1985).

These pieces of legislation, the demonstration projects sponsored by the Office of Special Education and Rehabilitative Services, the work of a number of private and university-based organizations promoting greater employment opportunities for persons with handicaps, and a generally increased awareness of the capacity for employment of people with developmental disabilities have led to an expanded range of employment options in the community. A variety of supported work and transitional employment programs have been important new initiatives (Beziat & Pell, 1985; Campbell, 1985; Chernish, Britt, Nutter, & Sakry, 1985; Conley, 1985; Conley & Noble, 1985; Keraschsky et al., 1985; Kiernan & Stark, 1986), and are discussed more fully in Chapter 5.

Consideration of the economic factors affecting the availability and accessibility of developmental services must take into account the increased range of employment options, preferences, and circumstances of people with developmental disabilities. Those circumstances, of course, include many of those factors noted above, such as levels of demand for labor in the community, the types of work available, prevailing wages, and other aspects of the labor market that all workers face. However, people with developmental disabilities must also deal with other significant exogenous constraints that affect their economic behavior.

Income Maintenance and Employment

Despite the recent history of legislation in the area of vocational rehabilitation, employment is still largely incompatible with other major elements of community-based services. Conley, Noble, and Elder (1986) provide an excellent review of some of the major problems in the current services system with respect to employment. They point out that the various vocational rehabilitation, employment, income support, medical assistance, housing, and other services do not operate in the coordinated fashion of a system. Most notably, the income support (SSI and SSDI) and medical assistance

(Medicaid and Medicare) programs on which substantial portions of developmental services are based have strong biases and disincentives against employment.

The disincentives created by these programs operate in several ways. First, these programs create attitudes and habits that are prejudicial to work. In order to qualify for either SSDI or SSI and subsequently for Medicare or Medicaid, applicants for these programs must demonstrate that they cannot earn above the Substantial Gainful Activity (SGA) level currently set at $300 per month. This inability to earn at the SGA level may be established in either of two ways. If they have no prior earnings history, as one would expect of young persons moving from school to adult services, and if they have one of a long list of disabling conditions that have been established by the Social Security Administration (e.g., an IQ below 60), then their inability to earn above the SGA level is established. If they do not qualify on the basis of the listed conditions or if they have a history of substantial work, then they must convince the Disabilities Determination Unit of the Social Security Administration, on the basis of medical examinations and forms, that they are unable to work at an SGA level. The process of establishing eligibility may take from 2 months to a year. At the end of this time, many people have convinced themselves that they are unable to engage in substantial work.

It should be emphasized that few people outside the Social Security Administration believe that one can determine who can work and who cannot work on the basis of the type of disability or a medical examination. Not only are the factors determining employability far more complex but it is also becoming increasingly accepted that many people who receive income support could work if appropriate services were provided.

A second type of work disincentive arises because a return to work by persons on SSI or SSDI may result in little gain and sometimes a sharp decrease in income. This is particularly striking in the SSDI program where earnings above the SGA level ($300 per month) result in termination of benefits after a trial work period. Because many disabled people can find work only in low-paying jobs and because the average SSDI payment is 50 percent above the SGA level (and some beneficiaries receive far more), the potential for a substantial reduction in income as a "reward" for returning to work is clear. Not only would the beneficiary lose his or her SSDI payment but he or she would also have to pay taxes and incur normal and sometimes disability-related work expenses. In addition, persons who lose their SSDI benefits will also lose their Medicare entitlement after 3 years.

Before 1981, persons on SSI lost their SSI payment and usually Medicaid if they returned to work at the SGA level or above after a 9-month trial work period. However, Congress enacted two 3-year demonstration projects for SSI recipients beginning in 1981 that were subsequently extended to June 30, 1987 by the Social Security Benefits Reform Act of 1984. One of the demonstrations is generally referred to as the 1619 (A) demonstration. Under this program, SSI recipients who return to work are not always terminated from the program after the trial work period. Instead they are allowed up to an $85 earnings and income disregard. After this disregard, benefits are reduced by $1 for each $2 of earnings. Federal benefits cease only when monthly earnings reach the federal breakeven point. For an individual in 1986 with no other income, this amount is $757 (calculated as the $85 disregard plus two times the benefit amount for an individual, which was $336 per month). Some states that pay SSI supplements continue to supplement beyond the federal breakeven point.

The other demonstration is usually referred to as the 1619 (B) demonstration. It provides extended Medicaid benefits to SSI beneficiaries who return to work provided that they continue to be disabled, require medical coverage in order to work, and their income falls below a threshold level.

A third type of work disincentive arises because most people, whether disabled or not, seek income security. Income security is a reason why unions bargain for seniority provisions in contracts, university professors seek tenure, and high-level executives in large corporations insist on "golden parachutes" when they accept jobs. Correspondingly, some persons with disabilities can be expected to resist sacrificing secure public support for jobs that are often low-paying and insecure.

Changes in the SSI and SSDI programs since 1980 have reduced but have not eliminated work disincentives (Conley et al., 1986). Persons on SSDI still face both a potentially large loss of income if they return to work and the eventual loss of Medicare benefits. Although the 1619 (A) and 1619 (B) demonstrations will probably be extended or made permanent in 1987 when the current authority for these programs ends, until this is done, the lack of certainty about the future of these programs is itself a work disincentive. In addition, other operating procedures in the 1619 (A) and (B) programs, such as limits on the amounts of earnings that recipients can receive and still remain eligible for Medicaid and the risk of losing 1619 (A) benefits permanently if earnings exceed the breakeven point temporarily, create work disincentives.

In addition to the perverse dynamics that exist between income support, work, and medical assistance, the housing of a person with developmental disabilities is a crucial element in the matrix. Many disabled persons live in community residences largely supported by the SSI payments of its residents. They may face the loss of a place to live if they become ineligible for SSI because of their increased income from work, and then they may lose their job.

The employment programs outlined above may serve to enhance disabled persons' more normal involvement in community life through work. However, these programs or employment do not necessarily eliminate the need for or desirability of congregate or supportive living arrangements for these individuals. Once again there is a dysfunctional relationship between work and another crucial element of community-based developmental services.

Summary

The economic behavior of persons with developmental disabilities, largely through their employment, is an increasingly important consideration in their access to developmental services and the overall structure of those services in a community. Not only are many individuals with disabilities successfully employed, but through a variety of incentives and programs, even larger numbers of more severely disabled people are working in traditional sheltered workshops, supported work programs, and in competitive employment. Despite some reforms to reduce work disincentives, people with developmental disabilities who seek employment and enhance their earnings face powerful disincentives in the potential loss of income support, medical assistance, and housing. Conley has pointed out that the attitude of the disabled person toward work is a crucial factor in vocational success (1973). It is difficult to imagine how the employment of people with developmental disabilities can be sustained or increased to allow their fuller involvement in the economic life of the community and in participating in important choices about their own well-being in the face of the perverse dynamics between work and other components of community-based services.

FAMILIES OF DISABLED INDIVIDUALS
AND THE ECONOMICS OF DEVELOPMENTAL DISABILITIES

One of the key facts about the circumstances of people with developmental disabilities is that the overwhelming proportion of these individuals live with their families, not only as children but also as adults (Hauber, Bruininks, Hill, Lakin, & White, 1982). On the one hand, the role of the family in caring for a member with a disability has been a central issue in social policy for hundreds of years (Moroney, 1983). On the other hand, although family members are obviously key to the care of people with developmental disabilities, the focus on the reciprocal effects of the family and the disabled member in the field of developmental disabilities has been relatively recent (Bruininks, 1979; Dybwad, 1966; Farber, 1968; Horejsi, 1979). Even more recent has been the attention to the costs of caring for a developmentally disabled family member and its consequences (Agosta, Bradley, Rugg, Spence, & Covert, 1985; Boggs, 1979; Comegys, 1985; Conley, 1973; Montgomery, 1982; Perlman, 1983; Roth, 1979; Turnbull, Brotherson, & Summers, 1985). In this section of the chapter, the particular concern is how do families behave with respect to the costs of care, and what effect does that behavior have on the availability and accessibility of community-based developmental services. Specifically, what are the costs that families bear in the care of the disabled member? And, more important, how have these costs been allocated between families and society, and what changes have occurred that affect the availability and accessibility of community-based services?

Costs of Care

Conley's (1973) work was one of the first major attempts to address the costs of mental retardation. His analysis of the specific costs to families focused on the loss of the value of the homemaker services of women with mental retardation. He also examined opportunity costs incurred: what a caregiver (typically a mother) would earn if she was able to enter the work force instead of remaining at home to care for a retarded child. Boggs's (1979) examination of the economic factors in family care outlined many of the costs associated with the care of a disabled child, and more recently, Comegys (1985) reviewed the impact of those costs, e.g., physicians, medicines, therapists, special equipment and devices, special babysitting, and transportation). Agosta and his colleagues examined the costs of caring for a developmentally disabled family member in their survey of families in Virginia and found that the median "special costs" incurred by families was $1,100 per family per year (Agosta et al., 1985). That study also reported that 39 percent of the families surveyed had opportunity costs, including giving up a paying job (14.7 percent), not taking a job (19.9 percent), and refusing a job transfer or promotion (10.8 percent). Obtaining more information about the specific economic costs of family care will have an impact on public policy in this area. However, the costs are clearly high, and the question within the context of this analysis is how these costs affect the behavior of families, and how does that affect the availability and accessibility of developmental services?

Who Bears the Costs of Care?

One of the most important issues of social policy is the extent to which individuals, families, and society share in the costs of care of people with disabilities. Closely linked to that issue are the specific mechanisms of social policy that are used to assume the costs of caring for a disabled family member.

Historically, the overarching issue has been institutionalization. Although there are many important factors affecting a family's decision to place a developmentally disabled family member in an institution, that choice has traditionally been virtually the only avenue that allowed a family to transfer the cost of care to society at large.

Both the closing of public facilities and more severe constraints on admissions have made institutionalization of a developmentally disabled family member, especially a child, much less available. However, in many important respects, the choices available to families for minimizing the costs of care are still framed by the issue of institutionalization. Previously unavailable community-based programs are beginning to provide essential services to people with disabilities, and supports to parents that assist them in caring for that child at home are also becoming more widespread. Nonetheless, the care of a developmentally disabled family member at home is influenced by a set of peculiar and shifting incentives and disincentives.

Families and the Cycle of Services It has only been within the past 10 or so years that families who chose not to seek an out-of-home placement for their developmentally disabled child have been able to defray the costs of care through other mechanisms and approaches. One of the most important sources of funding has been Medicaid, which is a vehicle for public assumption of the costs of medical/clinical therapies required for a disabled family member. However, to be eligible for Medicaid, the family must qualify through a means test, which discriminates against lower middle- and middle-income families. For preschool children, usually no earlier than the age of 2, many states have assumed the costs of therapeutic and some related services, such as transportation, through their education systems. Other states, such as New York, have paid for substantial portions of therapeutic services for preschool children through general tax levies. Nonetheless, timely access to early intervention services and family supports is generally regarded as a very difficult problem. Of course, PL 94-142, the Education for All Handicapped Children Act, mandates a free, appropriate education (and related services) for children with handicapping conditions. A review of the costs outlined by Boggs (1979) and Comegys (1985) suggests that many of those direct economic burdens, "special costs," are not met by these public programs. Perhaps as disabled children reach school age, the opportunity costs incurred by caregivers may be somewhat alleviated as they are able to seek employment during school hours. However, the relief from the costs of care provided by school programs is only temporary. At age 22, family members with developmental disabilities may again become a burden for their families as their access to day programs is no longer statutorily mandated, and families must seek an opening in a day program.

Family Support Services Recently, family support services have become more available as a mechanism to assist families to keep a family member at home. Although family support services are discussed more thoroughly in Chapter 5, it is important to point out some important facts about these services that affect a family's options. First, although the overwhelming majority of people with developmental disabilities live at home and will likely never seek institutionalization, much of the justification for the development of family support services and the eligibility criteria for them are based on prevention of institutionalization (Castellani, 1985). Second, these services were initially established as placement support services to ensure appropriate support services in the community for people who had been deinstitutionalized, and many of these support services are still focused on those individuals, rather than those who never were institutionalized (Castellani, 1985; Gollay et al., 1978; Commission on Quality of Care for the Mentally Disabled, 1984a). Finally, family support services have often been limited to the families of disabled persons already enrolled in routine day and residential services and are available largely through the organizations that provide those regular services (Castellani, Downey, Tausig, & Bird, 1986).

Families who choose to care for a disabled member at home face uncertain, incomplete, and perversely cyclical assistance from society for the care of that person. If families meet the means test of Medicaid, are fortunate enough to live in a state that provides in one way or another substantial preschool services, or have their own resources, they can bear the costs of care for a disabled preschool child. When the child reaches school age, the calculus changes as mandates for direct and related services create a different economic environment for the family. When that family member "ages out" of school programs, the family then faces a largely new set of economic issues. They again absorb many of the costs of care that had previously been provided through the school program, and most important, they are faced with negotiating for services in an environment without the statutory mandates within which they operated for the previous 16–18 years.

Tax Policy as a Vehicle for Family Assistance

There are a variety of current initiatives and proposals that will increasingly affect the capacity of a family to make choices about programs and services. Tax policy, which has come under increasing scrutiny, is a set of mechanisms that provide families caring for a disabled family member both relief from their financial burden and a wider range of choice in programs and services. A family's federal income tax deduction allows them to defray many of the costs of special equipment, adaptive devices, medical and dental services, pharmaceuticals, and other "special costs" of care noted above (Agosta & Bradley, 1985b; Perlman, 1983). Tax credits, particularly for child and dependent care, are another means of allowing families to obtain access to home care and special child care for a developmentally disabled member (Perlman, 1983).

In addition to typical exemptions, credits, and deductions, recent changes in the tax law have provided other avenues of financial relief for families with a disabled member, as well as increasing their options in accessing services and resources. Agosta and Bradley (1985c) review the "Cafeteria Benefit Plan" enacted in the Tax Reform Act of 1984 by which employers can offer their workers choices between taxable income or fringe benefits that are excludable from gross income. They point out that the flexible spending arrangements allowed under this plan (Benefit Bank Accounts and Zero Balance Reimbursement Accounts) are attractive options for families with a disabled member who may require services and expenses covered under a comprehensive fringe benefit package (Agosta & Bradley, 1985c, pp. 172–173).

There are, of course, a variety of problems associated with the use of tax policy, and the benefits vary greatly with the family's income, occupation, and need (Agosta & Bradley, 1985c; Perlman, 1983; Piachaud, Bradshaw, & Weale, 1981). Nonetheless, the use of tax policy to provide additional resources and options for families caring for a developmentally disabled family member not only provides "tax expenditures" for these families but also gives them a greater flexibility to choose services outside traditional institutional and organizational bounds.

Insurance, Disability Allowances, Subsidies, and Vouchers

Private insurance can relieve the financial burden of caring for a disabled member (Agosta & Bradley, 1985c; Bishop, 1981; Kane & Kane, 1978). However, although private insurers find that home care is less costly than institutional care, in general, private insurance for the costs of long-term care is both relatively unavailable and extremely expensive.

Moroney (1981) has argued for the adoption of a universal family disability allowance similar to those used in many European countries as a way to rationalize the many inconsistent and often conflicting ways in which current social policy addresses the financial burden of the family and its capacity to make choices about the services it needs for its disabled member. That issue of a family's ability to make choices is the basis of the use of direct cash subsidies and vouchers in several family support services programs.

Cash subsidies and vouchers are a major alternative to the direct provision of services by a government agency or contract organization. These mechanisms provide families with substantially greater flexibility and latitude in selecting service options for themselves and their disabled family members. They do not, however, appear to yet constitute any significant proportion of the funds available for community-based developmental services, although Bird (1984a), as well as Agosta, Jennings, and Bradley (1985), reported that several states have instituted the use of cash subsidies and/or vouchers in family support programs. Zimmerman (1984) has also reported the results of a family subsidy program in Minnesota that was intended to assist families to prevent out-of-home placements of a developmentally disabled member. Nonetheless, to the extent to which they are employed, the choices of families will increasingly create market-like conditions as they use the flexibility of subsidies and vouchers to purchase services from a wider array of vendors.

Conclusion

The family plays a central role in the care of people with developmental disabilities. The family's role was historically limited to the watershed choice of institutionalizing a disabled member or bearing virtually the entire burden of care at home. The introduction of a variety of public programs, such as Medicaid and the Education of All Handicapped Children, has had an enormous impact on a family's capacity to keep a disabled member at home, but these and other public programs and services still involve income, age, and other eligibility criteria that make their use by families rather problematic. Tax policies, private insurance, and other mechanisms provide some financial relief to families and a range of options beyond publicly provided or purchased services. Finally, family support services, albeit still bounded by institutionalization and direct provision of services by large organizations, are growing in importance as another avenue that gives families greater direct support and, especially with cash subsidies and vouchers, greater flexibility in the use of those resources.

In considering the impact of these various programs, services, and initiatives, it appears that there is indeed important movement toward greater amounts of support and autonomy for families caring for a disabled member at home. Thus, it is likely that the behavior and choices of families seeking services and resources for the care of their disabled member will have an increasingly important effect on the availability and accessibility of family support services.

THE ECONOMICS OF SERVICE ORGANIZATIONS

Deinstitutionalization and the creation of community-based services for people with developmental disabilities have brought about some of the most radical changes in human services in recent history. The organizational landscape of developmental services has been greatly altered. Services for people with developmental disabilities that were formerly available either in large state-operated institutions or in a very few small educational programs operated largely by parent groups are now provided through a myriad of state government, local government, private voluntary, and proprietary agencies.

Private voluntary and proprietary agencies have become especially important in providing community-based developmental services. Some attention has been devoted to the ways in which some agencies began to provide developmental services (Rothman & Rothman, 1984) and the relationships among provider agencies at the local level (Elder & Magrab, 1980; Savage et al., 1980). These and related issues are discussed in Chapter 5. However, despite the increasing awareness of the crucial role played by private agencies in providing developmental services, there has been little attention paid in the literature to the economics of these private organizations in the developmental services field, although Gilbert's work (1983) does examine the implications of "welfare capitalism" in the social welfare area. Bradley's work (1981) is one of the very few analyses that shows a broad appreciation of private organizations' relationship to other aspects of providing developmental services. The fiscal stability of these organizations and their capacity to acquire capital, cope with rising labor costs, market their products, and function in a complex three-sector economy while providing habilitative services to their clients are crucial issues affecting the availability and accessibility of community-based organizations.

The economic problems faced by private organizations have become of increasing concern to administrators and policy-makers. The identification and assessment of the important economic factors affecting these organizations should be integrated into a comprehensive framework for considering the availability and accessibility of community-based developmental services. Although there are a large number of concerns and problems in this area, this section focuses on three sets of issues that have emerged as major factors affecting the private service organizations and the availability and accessibility of developmental services: 1) managing the rapid growth and changes in the role of voluntary agencies, 2) the problems of operating a habilitation business, and 3), the impact of private developmental service organizations on local economics.

From Advocacy to Business: Managing the Rapid Growth of the Private Provision of Developmental Services

The first important fact about the private organizations that provide developmental services is their existence and significance in the field. A review of the literature dealing with community-based developmental services focuses largely on the various funding sources and mechanisms, on the one hand, and the specific services themselves, on the other. Aside from a few analyses of the problems of access to governmental generic services, there is virtually no recognition that a substantial amount of community-based developmental services are indeed provided by private organizations. That is, there seems to be little appreciation of the importance of the organizational context of the developmental services. Yet, these agencies, especially those in the private sector, are more than neutral conduits that transform funds into services.

Another significant feature of these organizations that is important to their economic viability is the relatively short period of time that they have played a major role in providing developmental services. The fact that many voluntary agencies have been radically transformed from small parent advocacy groups to multimillion dollar service-providing enterprises in a few short years seems to have implications for the viability and effectiveness of these agencies. The author's interviews with a wide variety of private agency directors, association representatives, parent-advocates, and state and local government administrators identified a group of factors that are important to the stability and viability of these private agencies.

One of the first concerns that was raised in these interviews was the problem presented by the lack of or confusion about the definition of the role of many private voluntary agencies. These agencies had previously been primarily parent support groups, vehicles for advocacy for additional and improved services for their family members, and occasionally, operators of small educational programs. Many of these agencies became large community-based providers of residential and habilitative services as states looked to them to take on those functions in order to facilitate deinstitutionalization. The rapid movement from small parent advocacy organizations to large service providers has created an overall ambiguity between advocacy and service provision that has led some of these organizations to spin off the service provision component into a separate and distinct agency. For many agencies that have not done so, there has been an increasing tension, if not divisiveness, between the parents who previously dominated (indeed operated) the organization and the large numbers of professionals and (occasionally unionized) service employees who now operate the programs. This tension has led to management problems that affect the viability of some organizations (Cook, 1985).

In some instances, the ambiguity and tension noted above are often manifested in a board of directors that is not attuned to the evolving role of the agency and does not embody the expertise, range of experience, and community representativeness that is usually associated with successful multimillion dollar human service agencies, which is what these organizations have become. Boards of directors that represented the specific interests of parents and were oriented toward advocacy are not necessarily suited to defining the role, setting the directions, and overseeing and supporting the operation of large and complex service-providing agencies. A number of private agencies have foundered because their boards of directors did not know of or were incapable of dealing with asset management and operational problems that should have been within their purview (Commission on Quality of Care for the Mentally Disabled, 1984a).

Many private agencies providing community-based developmental services are not solely MR/DD specific, but rather serve a wide variety of people with mental and physical handicaps. Other agencies, such as sectarian social service agencies, provide an even broader range of human and social services of which developmental services may be a relatively small proportion of their overall mission. Still other agencies (e.g., local and state ARCs) have been involved with developmental disabilities for a long time and have only recently assumed a service delivery role; some agencies have only been established recently to provide community-based services to people who were being deinstitutionalized.

The complexity of an agency's developmental services program has an important effect on its management. Regulations, funding sources, eligibility criteria, operational guidelines, and other important elements differ from program to program. Agencies that operate ICF/MRs, other community residences, sheltered workshops, and family support service programs are involved in a much more complex management environment than agencies that operate a single program.

The problems of boards of directors are mirrored at the level of agency management. Usually, agency directors and top administrative staff are human service professionals who have risen through the ranks. Although most directors' own expertise, knowledge of programs, and ability to learn management skills have enabled them to become capable executives, a sufficiently large number of private agency managers have not been successful; during the author's interviews several key informants, including association representatives, indicated that this poor leadership is a problem threatening the viability and stability of many organizations. Labor relations, cash and asset management, marketing, product selection, and capital acquisition are among the major problems facing directors of developmental service agencies, and yet these are not skills associated with human service professions (Bryce, 1985). Indeed, one national association director saw this problem of agency management as so crucial that management training courses and recruitment of executive directors from private industry have become two of the highest priorities of that association.

The problems of private agency management are only partially a factor of the expertise of the executives. Private agency management faces especially difficult problems. One of the most pervasive, yet largely unacknowledged, problems is the newness of the agencies. That is, the experience of a large number of private organizations providing a full range of residential, habilitative, and support services to people with developmental disabilities is so recent (either with the service, the clientele, or both) that virtually every problem of service development, administration, and operations that emerges is a new problem. There does not exist a long-standing organizational or industry-wide body of expertise and experience that provides routine guidelines for addressing problems. As a result, problems tend to become crises. What might be routine difficulties in organizations and industries in other sectors may threaten the very existence of the agency. It is difficult to measure the precise impact of this factor, but its importance in this area is often overlooked and underestimated.

A related concern noted by several association representatives and private voluntary agency executives is the relative absence of and reluctance to acknowledge a concept of a developmental services "industry." As suggested above, the movement from advocacy to service provision has been troublesome for some organizations. It seems that the suggestion that private, particularly voluntary, service providers should think of themselves as part of an industry is especially repugnant to many professionals in the field. Yet, despite the existence of statewide and national associations representing their interests, representatives of these groups almost universally point to the reluctance of private voluntary organizations to act more collectively and aggressively as an industry in matters of regulation, rate-setting, and other relationships with federal, state, and local governments that affect the economic well-being of these agencies. Of course, as Lowi (1979) and others have shown, provider rather than consumer interests tend to predominate in government-industry provider councils, advisory groups, and other such formal vehicles that trade associations tend to promote. Thus, the fundamental tension between advocacy and service provision that exists in many of these organizations serves to weaken their economic viability by inhibiting an unalloyed pursuit of the organization's self-interest.

At a more operational level, private organizations face a number of management problems peculiar to doing a large share of their business with governments. It is not unusual for a private agency in New York State to have 20 separate sources of income, which can include separate federal, state, and local government funding streams. Each funding source typically has separate regulations, eligibility criteria, funding mechanisms, reporting requirements, financial management, and operational guidelines. In addition to the enormous problems this creates for private agency management, the private agency doing business with a variety of government and private, such as United Way, programs finds itself often dealing in different and overlapping fiscal years. In New York State, for example, a private agency may commonly operate in separate federal, state, county, school district, and municipal fiscal years (Vandernoot, 1984). One analysis recently identified 10 separate reporting periods for 26 separate programs (Schielke, 1984). Under these and related circumstances financial management has been the primary source of economic instability for a number of private agencies.

A number of studies of the economics of sheltered workshops have indicated that management problems seriously affect the economic viability of these important community-based services (Conley, 1973; Conley & Noble, 1985; Noble, 1985; Stoikov, 1970). Poor product selection, pricing problems, inefficient work scheduling, and lack of attention to business-like marketing techniques have also been identified as management problems that compound the already substantial structural difficulties faced by sheltered workshops and private service agencies in general (Beziat & Pell, 1985).

In addition to the problems caused by the limited experience of private organizations operating large-scale community-based developmental services, a number of specific and important economic factors and dynamics affect the status of these organizations. In the following sections, a framework within which some of the important issues can be addressed is provided.

Private Organizations and Developmental Services

One of the first problems that must be faced when considering the economics of private developmental services organizations is that relatively little is known about the ways in which these organizations function. As White has pointed out, there is a need to "develop an overall theory of the behavior of nonprofit firms analogous to the theory of profit maximization for for-profit firms or the theories of staff or budget maximization behavior recently proposed for public sector bureaucracies" (1981b, p. 3). A second major issue is the role of the nonprofit organization in a three-sector economy in which governmental, nonprofit, and for-profit organizations all share or compete for a portion of the market (Weisbrod, 1975, 1977; White, 1981a, 1981b; Young, 1981). For instance, private voluntary organizations are very dependent on government grants and contracts for a major portion of their income, but must sell goods and services in the market for another substantial percentage of their income (Salamon & Abramson, 1982; White, 1981b). Indeed, this is the crux of what virtually all private agency, especially sheltered workshop, executives see as the problem of providing habilitative services and surviving as a business. One can best assess their problems by examining the economic contexts within which private organizations function: the controlled governmental environment, the semipublic world of rehabilitation facilities, and the private market.

The Private Agency in the Public Sector The private service organization operates in such a tightly controlled environment at all levels of government that it is difficult to describe the activities in terms of a public-private sector relationship. In many respects the private organization functions more like a governmental subsidiary than a private independent contractor. Market entry is typically closely controlled through such mechanisms as certification of an agency's fitness to provide developmental services and issuance of operating licenses that usually involve stringent physical plant standards, such as fire safety, and often stipulate numbers, types, and qualifications of staff, as well as detailed service program requirements. Medicaid-funded services are often characterized as involving the "three-legged stool" of certified providers, approved services, and eligible clients. Indeed, a private agency's access to clients is often tightly controlled by state government. Once in the market the price that a private agency receives for its services is determined by complex rate-setting processes for various types of programs. Indeed, the final price may actually be a composite of several rates. The amount of income for a community residence, for example, may be determined by a combination of the residents' SSI, SSI state supplementation, and a community residence rate that is based on a formula that takes previous reimbursement patterns, levels of staffing, and client characteristics into account. Despite individual agency and provider association activities, it is clear that the price paid for developmental services is largely stipulated by government and is not a result of a contractor's bid or a negotiated settlement that may characterize government-private sector relations in other areas. Thus, although they are ostensibly private entities, organizations providing community-based developmental services usually find that their ability to do business (enter the market), define the services they will provide, select their clientele, and set a price for their services is so highly constrained by government regulation and rate-setting that their definition as private economic actors seems unwarranted from that perspective. However, an examination of other important aspects of their service provision to people with developmental disabilities suggests that they do indeed operate in the environment of risk that tends to characterize the private sector.

As pointed out earlier, the rapid growth of community-based developmental services, especially those provided through private voluntary organizations, has masked a number of underlying problems that may affect the availability and accessibility of services through these organizations. On the one hand, many community-based developmental services were established by private voluntary agencies using a variety of startup and new development types of funding for which the agency or program no longer qualifies or which are now generally unavailable. Moreover, several states used Title XIX Medicaid funding for creation of Intermediate Care Facilities, and this funding stream has become increasingly problematic as a source of support for continued development. In addition, overall public funding for developmental services has plateaued. In general, private voluntary organizations that provide community-based developmental services seem to have reached a point at which some of the underlying economic problems and anomalies in this sector are becoming more evident and must be examined for their impact on the availability and accessibility of developmental services through these organizations.

Many private voluntary agencies are multimillion dollar enterprises that operate large numbers of day and residential programs and own many residences, workshops, clinics, other program sites, equipment, and vehicles—its capital in the classic sense. Under most state nonprofit corporation statutes, nonprofit firms are not prohibited from generating net revenues nor from accumulating those net revenues (profits) over time, as long as they do not distribute their profits to anyone as outside equity interests (Hansmann, 1980; White, 1981b). These accumulated net revenues may be used in a variety of ways. They are an especially important source of funds for recapitalization of buildings and equipment, and they may provide the agency with the fiscal capacity to smooth temporary gaps in cash flow or to act as seed money for new projects. Despite the statutory latitude available to nonprofit firms in general, state and local government rate-setting and contractual relationships with private voluntary agencies providing developmental services typically require these agencies to operate on a year-to-year contractual basis. Moreover, rate-setting formulas and purchase of service contracts do not allow for, and indeed prohibit, the accumulation of net revenues. Fundraising, sales, and other private agency revenues outside those funding streams are used as offsets against the total amount of funds that are eligible for government cost-sharing. One important effect of these government-private organization relationships is to leave those agencies in a position of year-to-year fiscal dependency. This is particularly true for agencies that only provide developmental services, have only been in existence or operating as a service provider for a relatively few years, have little or no endowment, and do not have parent organizations as a source of backup financial support. As a result, a substantial number of private voluntary organizations are placed in financially vulnerable positions and with little or no capacity to weather variations in cash flow or to recapitalize from within. In terms of recapitalization, private agency executives point to the decreasing amounts of funds available from the federal and state governments for capital expenditures, the extreme reluctance of banks to lend to organizations in the financial position noted above, and the lack of any widespread impact of various innovative capital pooling and similar schemes (Baldwin & Bishop, 1984; Shulman & Galanter, 1976). These are important constraints on the ability of private organizations to maintain the quality of their physical plants, to expand, and to purchase new equipment for both clinical and sheltered workshop programs.

In interviews with the author, several private agency executives and provider association representatives also maintained that allowances for administrative overhead in contracts for such programs as family support services were usually insufficient to cover the actual costs of administering them. Thus, larger, more well-established agencies typically absorbed the generally estimated 15 percent shortfall and/or transferred the costs to programs with more generous reimbursement for overhead. One effect of this situation, it was pointed out, was that small, newer agencies with less resources or capacity to absorb unreimbursed costs are either discouraged from participating in some programs or find that the costs become excessive.

Labor cost is another major problem that affects the business of habilitation and the economic stability of private voluntary agencies. The problem is relatively straightforward. In many states community-based developmental services are provided by both public and private agencies, and even where public agencies do not provide community-based services, they operate in close functional and/or geographic proximity to private agencies. In the developmental services field and in most other human services, public employees typically earn substantially greater salaries and fringe benefits than those earned by comparable employees of private agencies. This substantial salary and wage differential creates a great deal of staff turnover in private agencies as their employees routinely leave for public positions as they become available. The costs of retraining are difficult to measure, but are nonetheless an important concern. Of more pressing concern for private agencies is the pressure for salary and wage increases from their employees who have immediate evidence of salary and benefit disparities. One recent study by an association of private agencies serving people with mental disabilities reported salary differentials of 53–80 percent between state and voluntary agency community residence supervisors (McCrea, personal communication, 1985). Other studies have shown similarly large disparities (O'Neill, 1984; Oregon study, 1985), and there have been a number of proposals for government support to achieve or move toward wage parity between public and private sectors (Brancato, 1985).

In the absence of formal arrangements to achieve wage parity, staff turnover, the competition to recruit desirable professional and direct care staff, and unorganized and increasingly unionized demands for salary and wage increases have resulted in a larger labor cost in private agencies. Rate-setting formulas and budget-based contracts with state and local governments have allowed the absorption of some of these labor costs. However, the general slowdown in the increases in public funding for developmental services, as well as the increasing use of caps and block grant mechanisms, suggests that the ability to pass along increased labor cost will diminish, and these cost increases will become a larger threat to the financial stability of private agencies.

From one perspective, private voluntary agencies function within a tightly controlled fiscal environment. Dependence on federal, state, and local government grants, reimbursements, and contracts that are relatively short-term, provide little or no ability to accumulate income, and limited access to capital makes these organizations financially vulnerable. As government contractors providing the full range of developmental services to individuals for whom the federal and state governments have traditionally assumed a major responsibility, private agencies have seemingly operated with the implicit understanding that the government will ultimately rescue them from the consequences of the inherent economic anomalies of their situations, the effects of factors over which they exercise little control, and mismanagement. Indeed, in many instances this has occurred. However, the number of private agencies that have foundered, as well as the number that barely survive but with a capacity to provide services efficiently and effectively that is impaired by their poor financial condition, should indicate that the issues raised here are crucial to the economic viability of this sector and the availability and accessibility of community-based services.

The Habilitation Business: Sheltered
Workshops and Supported Employment

The economic problems affecting private developmental services agencies are most apparent when one considers those activities that are operated to generate income while attempting to achieve service program objectives, particularly sheltered workshops, which are by far the largest adult service component of community-based developmental services (Campbell, 1985). Private organizations that operate rehabilitation facilities—sheltered workshops and/or the variety of programs that fall under the term "supported work"—face a set of problems that are peculiar to the economic twilight zone they occupy between government subsidy and the private market. They face both problems that are specific to the anomalous situation of these programs and troublesome management problems, such as labor costs and access to capital. In addition, the growth of supported work programs has created problems for traditional sheltered workshops and private agencies that operate these programs.

Sheltered, supportive, and other employment programs for people with developmental disabilities have received substantial attention from economists and other analysts who have examined costs and benefits (Conley, 1965, 1973, 1985; Conley & Noble, 1985; Hill & Wehman, 1983; Kimberly, 1968; Noble, 1985; Thornton, 1985). Underlying these analyses of the economic issues is the fundamental philosophical question of the relative needs for and relationships between habilitation and work (Campbell, 1985). Although Conley (1973) and others have shown that substantial proportions of people with developmental disabilities do indeed work and even larger numbers can do so, the economic viability of the private voluntary agency operating a sheltered workshop rests on an often precarious fiscal balance between income from several governmental sources and from market activities. Figure 3.2 shows the major sources of income of a typical sheltered workshop serving people with developmental disabilities in New York State.

The fiscal balance is a precarious one because the sheltered workshop is faced with conflicting pressures. On the one hand, the Rehabilitation Comprehensive Services and Developmental Disabilities Amendments of 1978 (PL 95-602) requires state vocational rehabilitation facilities to give priority to clients with severe mental and physical handicaps. On the other hand, it should be obvious that the fiscal viability of the sheltered workshop depends in large measure on more productive clients who allow the workshop to compete for and complete contracts. It is not uncommon for a traditional sheltered workshop to have several hundred clients, scores of employees, and millions of dollars invested in its physical plant and equipment (New York State Association for Retarded Children, 1985).

The movement toward supported work programs has increasingly put pressure on sheltered workshops to move their more productive clients into these new programs. Although the philosophical and fiscal incentives for supported work programs have encouraged many rehabilitation facilities to develop more such pro-

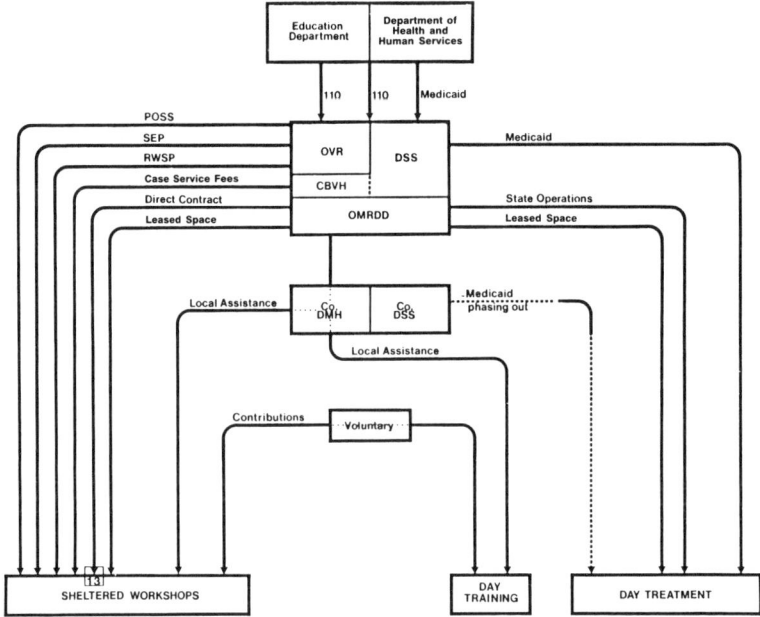

Figure 3.2. Funding streams for day programs. 110 = Section 110 funding, Vocational Rehabilitation Act; CBVH = Commission for the Blind and Visually Handicapped (NY); DMH = Department of Mental Hygiene (NY); DSS = Department of Social Services (NY); OMRDD = Office of Mental Retardation and Developmental Disabilities (NY); OVR = Office of Vocational Rehabilitation (NY); POSS = Purchase of Service System; RWSP = Rehabilitation Workshop Support Program (discontinued); SEP = Sheltered Employment Program. (*Source:* Bird, 1984b; reprinted with permission).

grams, it is also clear that these conflicting fiscal dynamics present substantial economic problems for many traditional sheltered workshop agencies that face the prospect of surviving with a more disabled clientele, relatively inadequate governmental funding, and a decreased capacity to compete in the private market. One analyst who has been involved in employment programs at the federal and state level has suggested that the militancy of some of the advocates of supported work in attacking traditional workshops for "backwardness" has resulted in counterproductive infighting among rehabilitation service providers (Noble, 1985).

In addition to the problems noted above, several analysts have also pointed out that many sheltered workshops suffer from severe management and structural problems that seriously impair their ability to survive. Many workshops are poorly managed (Beziat & Pell, 1985; Conley, 1973, 1985; Conley & Noble, 1985). In addition to the lack of qualified production managers, other management problems result in poor product selection, pricing, and marketing, which adversely affect the fiscal viability of these organizations. Because the clients of many workshops have similar disabilities, the range of goods and services that the workshop can produce is limited, and many workshops lack sufficient funds to purchase and maintain the equipment that would allow them to compete for more lucrative work. Moreover, Conley also notes that the small size of many workshops prevents economies of scale and results in the "inherent inefficiency of the sheltered workshop" (1985, p. 198).

A large number of sheltered workshops have overcome the problems outlined above and have become successful enterprises. National and state rehabilitation association leaders point to a number of traditional sheltered workshops that have dropped their explicit disability identification, and many workshops increasingly employ nondisabled workers. However, as well-managed, aggressive, and well-situated sheltered workshops produce competitive services and goods, enter new markets, and become successful business enterprises, they have produced a backlash from private for-profit businesses. Groups representing private for-profit businesses have argued that the tax-exempt status of nonprofit organizations and the various direct and indirect governmental subsidies enjoyed by these organizations give them an unfair advantage in the market (United States Small Business Administration, 1984). Nationally directed strategies for private for-profit businesses are underway to lobby state and local governments to eliminate these perceived advantages (Business Coalition for Fair Competition, 1985). Thus, the sheltered workshop sits in the position of economic vulnerability in its traditional position of "inherent inefficiency" and is under attack from the private for-profit sector when a more aggressive business-like stance produces unwanted competition.

The Business of Habilitation:
Developmental Services and the Private Sector

The private for-profit sector is an important component of community-based developmental services. This sector includes: 1) the small "Mom and Pop" element that has been a factor in community-based services for many years, 2) an increasingly important business segment, and 3) the relatively recent phenomenon of for-profit spinoffs of private voluntary agencies.

Profit-making spinoffs of private voluntary agencies are becoming more important to the economic survival and well-being of many agencies, especially as government subsidies and other support provide a smaller percentage of an agency's income (Meyers, 1985). In general there are three types of spinoffs. The first is the nonprofit organization that develops a product or service that can be best exploited through a profit-making entity that does not threaten the tax-exempt status of the parent private voluntary organization. A second type is the for-profit entity that allows the organization to take immediate economic advantage of its property; for example, selling the air rights or mineral rights on real estate owned by the parent organization. The third results from the situation in many states in which much of the community-based developmental services (both day and residential) are funded by Medicaid and effectively discourage access by middle-income individuals and families who are not otherwise categorically eligible for Medicaid. For-profit subsidiaries of private voluntary agencies have been organized to allow clients and families who can pay for services to gain access to them.

The so-called Mom and Pop providers of community-based developmental services have in many respects been the bulwarks of the for-profit sector for years. For the most part they have operated family care homes and larger community residences. Changing demographics, including a larger number of working women, a decreasing reliance on relatively unskilled labor on family farms, and smaller housing, have limited the possibilities of growth of these types of facilities. In addition, increasing costs of operation, such as are necessary to meet fire safety standards, have made this relatively small private proprietary sector more economically vulnerable.

The corporate segment of community-based developmental services has grown substantially in recent years and plays a large role in the availability and accessibility of these services in several states (Bradley, 1981; Welch, 1982). Privatization, the use of private for-profit businesses to undertake what had been traditional government-operated services, is a phenomenon that has been particularly important in recent years and has been encouraged by the Reagan administration (Gilbert, 1983; Hatry, 1983). Community-based developmental services are multibillion dollar activities and, where permitted, represent an important entrepreneurial opportunity. In addition to corporate operation of nursing homes and related residential facilities for people with developmental disabilities, large corporations, including Fortune 500 companies, have begun to provide a full range of day and residential services in some states. Moreover, some of these corporations include subsidiaries that provide equipment, supplies, and other consumables to the organizations delivering the developmental services. In the author's interviews, representatives of several national and state provider associations noted the growing size of corporate involvement in this area, but were generally unsure of its impact on the availability and accessibility of community-based services. Several professionals echoed the concerns about access of the poor and otherwise disadvantaged individuals to corporate-operated medical facilities, but there seems to be little, if any, concrete evidence whether there is indeed restricted access. A recent study in Minnesota indicated no significant differences in per diem rates between nonprofit and proprietary ICFs, but this does not directly address the question of how the auspices affect an individual's access (Minnesota Developmental Disabilities Program, 1983).

Summary

Current and enhanced availability and accessibility of community-based developmental services depend on the economic vitality of the organizations that provide those services. Changes in the private sector are very possible, if not likely. Private voluntary agencies that were brought into the delivery of substantial community-based services in several states during periods of large-scale deinstitutionalization and through a variety of financial and other incentives now find themselves facing an apparent diminished fiscal commitment on the part of the federal government and uncertainty as to state and local government support. In addition to several general economic problems, the traditional sheltered workshops that have constituted the largest day service component of these agencies' programs are caught between inherent inefficiencies, on the one hand, and pressures to move toward other models of service, such as supported employment, on the other. The small-scale private proprietary sector that had been providing community-based services for a number of years now finds itself economically vulnerable as more expensive regulations and formal operational guidelines make the costs of doing business on a "Mom and Pop" scale prohibitive. Finally, an emerging corporate sector in the delivery of community-based developmental services raises questions about the economic impact of these organizations in a three-sector economy, as well as the availability of services from large-scale profit-making service providers. Overall, the economics of service organizations should be an important part of one's consideration of the economics of developmental services.

OTHER KEY ACTORS IN THE
ECONOMICS OF DEVELOPMENTAL DISABILITIES

A comprehensive political economy perspective on community-based developmental services, takes into account all the actors with a significant impact on the availability and accessibility of these services. The economic interests of people with developmental disabilities, their families, and the private organizations that provide developmental services have already been examined. In the discussion of the socioeconomic environment of these services, the reciprocal impact of developmental services on the economic well-being of a community and their effect on property values was noted. In this section, the economic interests of employees of developmental service providers are discussed as a factor affecting the availability and accessibility of community-based developmental services.

Some attention has been given to the role of public employees in the process of deinstitutionalization (Conroy & Bradley, 1985; Rothman & Rothman, 1984). Generally, public employees and public employee unions have resisted the efforts to close and/or substantially reduce the size of large public institutions. Despite rationalizations focusing around concerns for the well-being of people with developmental disabilities in new community settings, it is evident that the prospect of the loss of jobs and the need to relocate have been important economic factors in this resistance. It is nonetheless important to recognize that tens of thousands of employees providing care and services to people with developmental disabilities have had, and are likely to continue to have, an important impact on the availability and accessibility of community-based services.

In New York State the issue of protecting a substantial portion of the public employee positions that would be otherwise abolished in the rundown of large institutions was addressed by establishing state-operated day and residential community-based services (Rothman & Rothman, 1984). The relocation of thousands of public employees to state-operated ICFs, community residences, and day programs has undoubtedly reduced a major part of the opposition to deinstitutionalization that might be otherwise expected.

The growth of supported work programs raises the prospect of change in the size and structure of traditional sheltered workshops. Although possible employee dislocations from these workshops would not approach the magnitude of the closure of large state institutions, they are nonetheless an issue to be taken into account in considering the promotion of work programs outside the traditional model.

In summary, the economic impact of deinstitutionalization and other significant changes on employees is substantial, and it is very likely that any actual or perceived threat to their well-being will be quickly translated into political and other opposition to change. That obviously affects the availability of community-based services and the ways they are arrayed. A comprehensive political economy perspective should take into account the economic interests of employees of developmental service providers.

CONCLUSION

This chapter has examined the questions of who pays for developmental services and what impact does that have on the availability and accessibility of those services in community settings. Public funding has been and will likely continue to be the major source of financing, and the description of the various public funding sources and mechanisms illustrates the problems that public funding presents for enhancing community-based services in a comprehensive and coordinated fashion.

This chapter has also attempted to go beyond the boundaries of public finance to show how other, more private, factors affect the availability and accessibility of community-based services. The discussion of the behavior of disabled persons and their families in seeking to maximize their benefits and minimize their costs should make us sensitive to the fact that we need to more appropriately account for their behavior. The traditional dependent roles played by or assigned to these actors are less typical of their behavior in community settings. Moreover, a wider range of employment opportunities for people with developmental disabilities, the increased use of vouchers, cash subsidies, and private insurance by families, and the emergence of new providers of developmental services tend to create more market-like conditions in the community. These market-like conditions and behaviors often seem to work at cross-purposes with various public funding mechanisms that were not designed with these factors in mind. Thus, one important conclusion of this chapter is that the community context of developmental services involves new actors (or the same actors) in new roles that are more similar to private economic activities and less similar to the behaviors on which many public finance mechanisms are predicated.

The second important conclusion of this chapter is that the role and impact of private (voluntary and proprietary) service organizations need to be incorporated into a framework for assessing the availability and accessibility of community-based developmental services. There has been virtually no attention paid in the professional literature to the organizations that play an important role in providing developmental services. The roles and relationships among government agencies and private organizations that developed during the last 10 years of rapid deinstitutionalization may no longer be appropriate. There is an increasing awareness among state and local government administrators, as well as the provider community, that many voluntary agencies face a myriad of economic problems that may be beyond their organizational and managerial capacity to solve. Moreover, these organizations face pressures from the environment and changes in government programs, particularly in the vocational area, that bring into question their long-term roles in providing community-based services. The emergence of corporate providers of developmental services has raised questions about the appropriateness of these types of organizations as service providers. Generally, there is an apparent reluctance on the part of advocates, providers, and other key actors in the field to recognize that the provision of community-based developmental services is a multi-billion dollar endeavor that necessarily involves large and complex private organizations, both voluntary and proprietary. Once again, it seems that the failure to take this stratum of actors adequately into account results in some measure from the absence of a perspective that recognizes their legitimacy as independent forces in a community-based political economy.

The importance of the community environment to the availability and accessibility of developmental services is another major observation of this chapter. In much of the professional literature, the community is seen as an unspecified good place to provide services. The plain fact is that communities vary widely: from rich to poor, urban to rural, sympathetic to hostile to disabled people, and in many other ways that positively and negatively affect the availability and accessibility of developmental services. The extent to which developmental services are merely located in or are actually integrated with and naturally arise from the community context depends on many factors that have not been addressed in considering the availability and accessibility of services. These need to be examined in large part because they deal with the fundamental issue of equity that lies at the core of our concern. This chapter has identified some of those key factors and has also noted that developmental services and communities should be viewed as involving reciprocal and often mutually beneficial relationships.

The notion of mutually beneficial relationships raises another important observation that should be incorporated into a comprehensive perspective on developmental services. That is, "every dollar of expenditure is someone's dollar of income." The public finance approach to developmental services focuses almost exclusively on expenditures. A broader economic perspective should carry with it an appreciation that the other side of expenditure is income. Perhaps unfortunately, the issue has been raised almost exclusively in the context of the displacement of employees of large institutions. The economic impact of developmental services on communities can be viewed positively as well. In any case, this political economy perspective should be important in evaluating both the benefits and costs of community-based developmental services.

Finally, and perhaps most important, the observations and conclusions made in this chapter about various political-economic dimensions, issues, and relationships should not obscure the fact that they involve fundamental questions of efficiency and equity. In a number of instances it was pointed out that broader-based and multiple mechanisms for the delivery of developmental services in communities create more market-like conditions for consumers and providers. From the consumers' perspective—both disabled people and their families—a greater range of choice may seem desirable, at least in the abstract. However, as Lindblom (1977) has noted, the marketplace does not do a very good job of distributing equity. In the context of community-based developmental services one should not necessarily assume that the introduction of a greater number of choices for consumers will be either efficient or equitable. The introduction of these mechanisms into imperfect markets may serve to exacerbate existing inequities in access or availability. The increased use of market-like mechanisms may also undermine the fiscal stability of existing service providers whose (already tenuous) economic well-being is largely based on negotiated contracts for services, rather than competition for clients in market-like contexts.

Another important aspect of the equity issue concerns the variations in communities noted above. There seems to be a basic assumption that people with developmental disabilities are entitled to comparable services anywhere they live in a particular state. Indeed, comparability ("statewideness") and entitlement stem from the great reliance on Medicaid-funded services in many states. In promoting service provision in community contexts, advocates must address the question of what degree of variation in availability and accessibility will occur because of the factors in the community environment, such as wealth, willingness, ruralness, and the like. More importantly, advocates must also consider what degree of variation will be acceptable and, if it exceeds certain boundaries, how to address inequities of availability and accessibility. These are fundamental issues of equity that underlie much of the discussion of reliance on community-based services and market-like reforms in the funding and delivery of developmental services.

In conclusion, the greater reliance on community-based services entails many complex and troublesome concerns that have not been heretofore faced in the developmental disabilities area. In many respects, a focus on the economics of community-based developmental services provides an important set of tools and an analytic perspective that will allow the field to deal effectively with many of those issues and problems.

4

Access to Community Programs
Who Is Served?

THE ISSUE OF WHO RECEIVES COMMUNITY-BASED SERVICES IS THE MOST central and probably most difficult problem facing the field of developmental disabilities. The number of people who need and/or demand developmental services, as well as their individual, situational, and demographic characteristics, has an enormous impact on the ways in which services are organized and funded. Of course, the ways in which services are currently organized and funded are the most significant factors affecting access to developmental services. Nonetheless, the implementation of community-based services expected to serve a broad base of people with developmental disabilities requires that one examine two basic dimensions of the issue of access. As expressed from the perspective of public and private funders, administrators, and providers, the question is: "Who's out there?" The second question is most often asked by advocates and those seeking access to services: "How does one obtain access to developmental services?" This chapter is organized around these two questions. The objective of the chapter is to show that the answers to these questions are ambiguous and involve a wide range of factors that have only recently been acknowledged and assessed.

WHO'S OUT THERE?:
EPIDEMIOLOGY AT THE POINT OF DELIVERY

It is important to remember that 20 years ago the answer to the question, "Who's out there?," was largely irrelevant to state and local government administrators. They were concerned almost exclusively with the thousands of individuals who were in large state-operated institutions, and the waiting list for the next vacant bed, with occasional special admissions through other channels, was the primary epidemiologic consideration. In the community, children with developmental disabilities were largely excluded from public classrooms, and small educational programs and workshops operated and funded by parent groups comprised the majority of community programs. Although this is obvious to students of the field, it is important to appreciate the fact that at the outset neither deinstitutionalization nor the education of all handicapped children required much operational consideration of the definition of developmental disability, the epidemiology of developmental disabilities, or clearcut and explicit eligibility criteria for access to services. In the past 10 years a substantial proportion—in many states virtually all—of the community services that have been established have been created to accommodate those thousands of individuals who were previously institutionalized. Thus, those issues have been deferred. It is now becoming apparent that the demands for service by: (1) people who have not previously been in institutions, (2) those aging out of special education programs, (3) those with disabilities other than mental retardation, (4) very young children with disabilities, and (5) others in the community environment, have forced advocates, analysts, and policy-makers to take more than an academic interest in these issues of definition, epidemiology, and eligibility criteria.

Concept of Disability

The concept of disability entails substantial tension between a medicalized perspective, on the one hand, and a broad range of political, economic, situational, and behavioral factors, on the other. In her history of disability policy, The Disabled State (1984), Deborah Stone shows the derivation of medical definitions of disability in contemporary society. The large increase in the number of beneficiaries of disability programs in the past 20 years, especially with difficult-to-assess mental disabilities, is an indication of the medicalization of many social problems. Of particular interest is her question, "Why are educational problems such as reading difficulties now labeled 'learning disabilities' and diagnosed by clinical teams?" (Stone, 1984, p. 12). Her analysis of the important linkages between work and disability leads her to conclude that a concept of disability based on clinical criteria is bound to fail. Stone argues that the clinical concept of disability was intended to place a tight boundary around needs-based distribution, but she states:

> The assignment of citizens into the work-based and need-based distributive systems remains a highly political issue which is not readily resolved by the creation of formal administrative schedules or the dele-

gation of decisions to the medical profession (or any other technical experts). Thus there is a constant struggle over the boundaries which manifests itself in shifting pressures for expansion and contraction of the disability category. (Stone, 1984, p. 140)

Stone sees those pressures coming from individuals applying for benefits, from professional and administrative gatekeepers who apply their own norms, and from high-level policy-makers (legislators, administrators, and judges) who make the general rules that design and redesign the boundaries. Stone's analysis of the definition of disability points out the historical relationships between work and need, the problems involved in the medicalization of the definition, and the fundamental political struggle that shapes the boundaries of the disability system.

Berkowitz, Johnson, and Murphy (1976) add another important dimension to the concept of disability by pointing out its social and economic elements. They, as does Stone, argue that medical and health-related definitions are not adequate guides to who is disabled. Their analysis of the demographic, income, and health characteristics of SSDI applicants and recipients leads them to view disability as a behavior, occurring as a result of the interaction between those variables and the transfer payments from the disability insurance program. This view not only broadens the definition of disability but also indicates that it is not a phenomenon, no matter how inclusive, that can be adequately defined without reference to the social welfare program to which it relates.

These and other analyses of the concept of disability provide an important context for the question of who is developmentally disabled. What Stone and Berkowitz, Johnson, and Murphy make explicit is that disability is an ambiguous concept, one that encompasses a variety of historical, medical, socioeconomic, and behavioral factors and one whose boundaries and application are the result of political processes. These factors are very important in the community context of developmental services.

Definition of Developmental Disabilities

The ambiguities and complexities in the concept of disability are compounded somewhat in identifying and defining the parameters of developmental disabilities. Clearly, the work of Berkowitz et al. (1976) leads to a definition of disability that is primarily functional. However, there are a number of problems in planning for services, establishing eligibility criteria, and implementing programs when the basic framework for identifying the target population consists of a categorical-functional approach with a limited operational experience.

One of the first issues of importance is which disabilities are identified as developmental. Mental retardation has, of course, been the predominant focus in the field, but federal and state legislation and practice have expanded the categories of developmental disabilities to encompass an increasingly wide variety of conditions. Prader-Willi syndrome, Tourette's syndrome, and multiple sclerosis, for example, have come within the framework of developmental disabilities (Sacks, Smull, & Beverely, 1985). The movement toward a functional definition must also be seen within the context of advocacy to include more types of disability within the general framework.

The 1970 Developmental Disabilities Service and Facilities Construction Act (PL 91-517) used a categorical definition that included mental retardation, cerebral palsy, epilepsy, and other neurological impairments occurring before the age of 18. In 1975 the Developmental Disabilities Assistance and Bill of Rights Act (PL 94-103) added autism to the categories.

It was not until the 1978 Rehabilitation, Comprehensive Services and Developmental Disabilities Act (PL 95-602) that the recommendations of the National Task Force on the Definition of Developmental Disabilities for a functional approach to the definition were incorporated into statute. That definition targets individuals with substantial functional limitations in three or more of the following major life activities: self-care, receptive and expressive language, learning, mobility, self-direction, capacity for independent living, and economic self-sufficiency. It focuses on chronicity, early onset, multiple impairment, and the need for ongoing interdisciplinary services (Kiernan, Smith, & Ostrowsky, 1986).

The functional definition of developmental disabilities addresses many of the problems in the medical and categorical approaches identified earlier. It requires a specific focus on each individual in order to determine whether that person meets the eligibility criteria, and that identification is intended to be linked to the services needed by that person to meet his or her functional deficits (Kiernan et al., 1986; Lakin & Hill, 1985). However, there has been great variation in approaches to measuring the various functional components of the definitions and little experience in its application (Kiernan et al., 1986; Lubin, Jacobson, & Kiely, 1982; Summers, 1981). An additional problem with the functional definition is that many people with substantial mental and physical deficits are functionally competent because of the timely provision of services, and for many people with a categorical disability, functional competence may be episodic, rather than chronic (Conley, 1985). Finally, the various elements in the functional definition are more oriented toward adult activities, so that very young children with developmental disabilities or delays may not be adequately addressed, especially because this area is characterized by vague definitions (Lessen & Rose, 1980).

In general, the functional definition of developmental disability provides the field with an individualized, need-based, and service-oriented approach toward the people who fall within its boundaries. However, the pressure to expand the categories to include people with disabilities that often have ambiguous and episodic manifestations and the lack of extensive experience in its application make the use of this functional definition for planning, funding, and establishment of eligibility criteria complex and difficult (Lakin & Hill, 1985).

Prevalence of Developmental Disabilities

The planning, funding, and implementation of community-based services that are more available and accessible to people with developmental disabilities must rest on some reasonable calculation of the number and characteristics of the individuals who have developmental disabilities. The most important statistic that provides a measure of the number of individuals for which services must be planned and provided is prevalence; that is the number of people in a population who have the condition or illness during a period of time (Stein and Susser, 1975). This statistic provides one element of the answer to the question, "Who's out there?," by indicating the number of individuals that should form the universe of those needing service.

Kiernan and Bruininks (1986) provide an excellent review of a number of studies of the epidemiology of developmental disabilities. This review, as well as their inferences from data on subgroups not usually encompassed in most studies, leads them to conclude that "a prevalence rate of 1.49% of the general population is realistic. Overall, the prevalence rate across all ages would be closer to 1.6%" (Kiernan & Bruininks, 1986, p. 35). Nonetheless, they do point to several problems inherent in the studies on which their estimate is based. Among the most important are the varied methodologies used in the studies, their being based on the categorical groupings used before the adoption of a functional definition, and the substantial variations reported by age, region, and setting (Kiernan & Bruininks, 1986).

Although the Kiernan and Bruininks analysis and estimate of a prevalence rate is well supported, their review nonetheless points to the conclusion that epidemiologists vary widely in their estimates of the number of people with developmental disabilities. Moreover, even the lower prevalence rates would indicate that there are substantially more people with developmental disabilities than are receiving developmental services in preschool, school, and adult programs. Finally, advocacy groups typically argue that many more individuals have developmental disabilities than are indicated by the estimates of epidemiologists or government planning offices (Aird, Masland, & Woodbury, 1984).

This brief review underscores two main problems facing analysts, advocates and policy-makers concerned with access to community-based developmental services. First, it is clear that there are substantially more people with relatively severe developmental disabilities living in the community than are now being provided developmental services. Second, although the use of a functional definition represents important advances on several dimensions, the expansion in the types of disabilities encompassed within the general statutory and operational frameworks and the variation and ambiguities in the definition do not provide a very clear picture of the types of individuals "out there" who are likely to seek access to services.

OBTAINING ACCESS TO SERVICES

The various aspects of the question of "Who's out there?" obviously are important to answering the question of "how does one obtain access to services?" This latter question is the most difficult to answer. It is almost immediately apparent to advocates, analysts, and policy-makers that abstract estimates of the number of people with developmental disabilities provide little more than a vague background to the factors that are significant predictors of access to services. There are difficulties in determining eligibility criteria for such structured services as ICFs/MR (Lakin & Hill, 1985); the problems are compounded when considering the less-structured services that are now emerging in community contexts.

The number of individuals who are potential clients does shape the ways in which eligibility for services is determined. However, there are several other important sets of factors that more immediately and significantly affect access. They include the types and levels of disability, an individual's service history, a variety of demographic characteristics, and such situational factors as a family's capacity and willingness to care for a disabled member at home. There are also a number of factors that significantly affect access that are external to the person with a disability and his or her family. Geographic location, access to transportation, the capacity of the local service system, and its history of service to people with developmental disabilities are especially important external factors. The structure of services, including the auspice of the provider agencies and the extent to which services are aggregated in agencies, is another important consideration. Finally, the degree to which services are mandated judicially or through statute is of the utmost importance in determining how one obtains access to services. In this section of the chapter these factors are examined, and in particular, the interplay among demographic, situational, and service system characteristics is discussed.

Types and Levels of Disability

Developmental disabilities are defined both categorically and functionally. Although recent legislation has emphasized the functional approach, mental retardation as a categorical disability provides the most central definition for the field (Lakin & Hill, 1985). Persons with mental retardation are more likely to obtain access to services in the community than individuals with other developmental disabilities for several important reasons. First, the best predictor of access to community services is prior service, in an institution or from another provider, and the great majority of people placed out of large institutions have mental retardation. Second, although there has been considerable effort to operationalize a functional approach to developmental disability, the measurement of IQ remains the most widely used criterion for identification of a developmental disability (Lakin & Hill, 1985). Third, many community-based providers of developmental services have an explicit disability identification, and clearly those that serve persons with mental retardation and cerebral palsy, albeit not exclusively, provide the great majority of services. Not surprisingly, advocacy groups representing persons with disabilities other than mental retardation and cerebral palsy argue that there are not nearly enough programs designed to serve persons with those other disabilities (J. T. Farrelly, personal communication, January 13, 1986; P. A. Lilac, personal communication, 1986). Thus, although developmental disabilities comprise a number of separate disability types and a functional rather than categorical approach to need is emerging, the type of developmental disability still affects a person's ability to obtain access to services.

It is virtually axiomatic that people with the greatest need should have priority in access to services. However laudable that principle, one central problem is the difficulty of measuring the need for the types and levels of services that should be linked to various functional deficits (Grossman, 1983; Lakin & Hill, 1985; Meyers, Nihira, & Zetlin, 1979). The problems of identifying a developmental disability are especially difficult with very young children (Abeson & Zettel, 1977; Hayden, 1979). It is often difficult to assess a person's need independently of the services he or she may be receiving or without assessing a person's familial and social supports (Conley, 1985; Farber, 1968; Sussman, 1982). Moreover, the episodic or intermittent needs of many people with developmental disabilities who live in the community and do not receive regular services are not amenable to a relatively lengthy needs assessment process (Conley, 1973).

One recent approach to determining individuals' needs for services in Nebraska is described by Schalock and Keith (1986), who also outline some needs assessment approaches being implemented in other states. Keith and Ferdinand (1984) note that the need for services is not necessarily directly related to a person's level of disability and that a broader range of behavioral and situational factors must be taken into account. Fernald (1986) suggests that adoption of a diagnosis related group (DRG) approach to matching clients' needs to services should be explored. In general, these analyses make it clear that the type and level of an individual's developmental disability are often difficult to measure and are not themselves reliable criteria for how people obtain access to services.

Importance of Demographic and Situational Factors

Although the immediate focus of assessments of the need for service is on an individual's type and level of disability, a variety of demographic and situational factors play a key role in determining how one obtains access to services.

A person's *service history* is one of the most important factors affecting access to community-based developmental services. In many respects, community-based services have been and will likely continue to be developed to provide alternatives to large state-operated institutions. Persons being deinstitutionalized as a consequence of court orders, consent decrees, plans of compliance, and other social policy mandates and plans have been the primary group of clients for whom community-based residential and day programs have been established. A study of 135 family support services programs indicated that enrollment in an agency's routine day and residential programs was a primary eligibility criterion for access to that agency's family support program (Castellani et al., 1986). In New York State, concern about the inability or difficulty in gaining access to adult day services by individuals "aging out" of special education for handicapped children programs has resulted in state legislation that set up special procedures to facilitate the linkage between the service systems and special funding targeted for day programs for "aging out" individuals (New York State, 1984).

Service history has other peculiar effects, particularly for those individuals who are receiving services from other human service systems. A substantial number of people with developmental disabilities find themselves in mental hospitals, jails, and other inappropriate settings because community-based developmental services are not available (Rockowitz & Davidson, 1986). This suggests that once an individual becomes a client in another service domain, it is often difficult to gain access to services in the more appropriate developmental services system. Access to services is an incremental and cumulative process in many respects, and one's history of service use has an important impact on getting into developmental services.

Age is another crucial factor affecting access to developmental services. Early onset and chronicity are two of the most significant elements of the definition of a developmental disability, and developmental disability is lifelong for most affected individuals. Nonetheless, a developmentally disabled person's ability to gain access to services is highly dependent on his or her age and can vary substantially across certain age thresholds. Undoubtedly the most important thresholds are the ages for beginning and ending mandated education for children with handicapping conditions. Although this effect of age is widely recognized and discussed, other age-related influences on access to and use of services have only recently emerged.

Enhanced medical and related care has extended the life-span of many individuals with developmental disabilities. However, there is evidence that people with Down syndrome may exhibit signs of premature aging (Wisniewski & Hill, 1985), and in general, people with developmental disabilities face problems of aging from about their early fifties (Janicki & Jacobson, 1986). These problems often lead to increased needs for services at this time of life (Janicki & MacEachron, 1984; Janicki, Otis, Puccio, Rettig, & Jacobson, 1985; Seltzer, 1985; Seltzer & Selzer, 1985). An important related concern is the age of caregivers. As people with developmental disabilities reach their 40s and 50s, the increasing age and diminished physical and economic capacity of their parents and other caregivers can have an important effect on the disabled person's need for and use of services (Janicki, Krauss, Cotten, & Seltzer, 1986; Tausig & Epple, 1985).

Race and ethnicity affect a person's ability to gain access to developmental services. Several analyses have shown that persons from ethnic and racial minority groups are underrepresented in the developmental services system: as clients, as professionals, and as minority-operated provider agencies (Coleman. 1980; Dunlap, 1976; New York State Developmental Disabilities Planning Council, 1983; President's Committee on Mental Retardation, 1977; United States Department of Health and Human Services, 1981). Both overt discrimination and the problems faced by minority persons who are more likely to be economically and socially disadvantaged are seen as causal factors in this underrepresentation (Dana, 1981; Justice, O'Connor & Warren, 1971; Kernan & Walker, 1981; Reschly & Jipson, 1976). These problems include a language barrier, a lack of transportation, the relative absence of services in minority communities, and a lack of minority-operated agencies (Coleman, 1980; Eyman, Boroskin, & Hostetter, 1977; Reschly & Jipson 1976). In addition to specific barriers to access, there is also evidence to suggest that some ethnic and racial minorities—Hispanic and Asian groups being most frequently mentioned—are more inclined to rely on informal supports rather than formal services in caring for a member with a disability (Abad, Ramos, & Boyce, 1974; Aday, Chin, & Anderson, 1980; Blackwell, 1975; Sue & McKinney, 1975). In culturally and racially diverse communities the issues noted above have an impact on who receives services and constitute an important and difficult dimension of the problems of equity of access.

In Chapter 3 the effect of *wealth* on one's ability to gain access to developmental services was discussed at some length. An individual's or family's assets can be translated into transportation and a variety of other instruments that facilitate access to services. A number of individuals interviewed also suggested that a family's time and effort—commodities usually possessed by the economically advantaged—on behalf of a private agency's programs can be instrumental in enhancing a family member's ability to gain admittance to a program. It has also been suggested that outright monetary contributions to private agencies by families can enhance, if not ensure, acceptance of their family members into programs.

The role of a person's *family* as a crucial situational factor affecting access to services has become more recognized in the past several years. Since Farber's (1968) seminal work on the social context of mental retardation and the central importance of the family of the disabled person to his or her development, a number of analysts have explored various aspects of this area (Bruininks & Krantz, 1979; Gallagher & Vietze, 1986). The stress that the presence of a disabled member creates in a family has received substantial attention (Black, Small, Crites, & Sachs, 1985; Edgar & Heinowski, 1985; Gallagher, Beckman, & Cross, 1983; Horejsi, 1979; Perlman & Giele, 1983;

Wikler, 1986). Recently that attention has been directed toward the impact on the siblings of a disabled person (Edmundson, 1981; Simeonsson & Bailey, 1986). Conversely, the supports provided by a family structure have also been shown to be essential to the well-being of people with developmental disabilities (Farber, 1968; Frankfather, Smith, & Caro, 1983; Turnbull, Summers, & Brotherson, 1986). Many analysts argue that rehabilitation strategies should be designed to permit family members a larger role in the rehabilitation process (Berger & Foster, 1986; Sussman, 1982).

Although there is a growing body of literature that describes the importance of the family, its exact impact on a disabled person's need for and use of services is not always clear. Tausig and Epple (1985) examine the relationships among individual, family, and service system characteristics in the decision to seek out-of-home placements. They find that family structure is a crucial factor in risk of placement and describe several family profiles, including dual-career, families with loss of the primary caregiver, and older families, that distinctly increase the likelihood of placement. As the focus of concern turns toward the use of community-based developmental services, it is imperative that the role of the family be more carefully examined.

The important role of the family also adds another major dimension to the question of who is served. Family support services, which are relatively new, involve a new clientele for developmental services: fathers, mothers, and siblings of people with developmental disabilities (Castellani, 1985). This exponential increase in the number of people who seek access to services is likely to have an effect on the overall capacity of developmental services in a community and may ultimately affect the question of who gains access to services.

Where a person lives also has an important impact on his or her access to developmental services. The extent to which developmental services are available in a person's community and their location are significant factors affecting access. Transportation to work, day programs, and other services is often cited as a significant problem for people with developmental disabilities (Gollay et al., 1978; Kiernan & Ciborowski, 1985).

Environmental and Service System Factors

The effect of a person's sociodemographic characteristics on his or her ability to gain access to developmental services should be considered together with the effect of such environmental and service system characteristics as the capacity and structure of developmental services in a community, historical trends in developmental services, and the impact of statutory or judicial mandates.

Local *service system capacity* and structure are briefly discussed in Chapters 3 and 5. However, it is important to restate the obvious point that who is served depends in large measure on how many community-based developmental services exist. Many community-based services were established specifically for people being deinstitutionalized and/or target groups who are given priority for entry into the programs. The degree to which the local system of services is sufficiently large and targeted to meet the needs of people with developmental disabilities within the community alters the impact of the sociodemographic variables outlined above.

In addition to the capacity of the developmental services in a community, some *structural considerations* also affect who is served. There are a variety of types of developmental services, and often there are gaps between availability and need. Poor planning, the fiscal incentives to implement certain types of programs, such as ICFs/MR, and uncertainty about the numbers and types of clients in a community are among the major factors that can contribute to the establishment of community-based programs that do not meet the needs of the population (Human Services Research Institute, 1985a). ICFs/MR established to meet the needs of people being deinstitutionalized that have a large capacity and an absence of less clinically intensive vocational and other day programs in a community obviously limit the access of less severely disabled individuals.

Other structural factors, such as the *auspice of the provider agency*, may have an impact on who is served. Members of racial and ethnic minority groups may be inhibited from seeking access to agencies that they feel are not culturally or linguistically receptive to them. Many private voluntary agencies have a distinct cultural and religious identification that explicitly or implicitly inhibits access by disabled people from other groups. Another example of how certain structural factors affect access is in family support services. Many family support services are funded in part by local government, and one study of these services showed that access to these services was limited to the residents of the local government jurisdiction that provided the funding (Castellani et al., 1986). That same study showed that, in large multiprogram agencies, priority for one type of service was given to people who were enrolled in other programs operated by the agency. Thus, whether developmental services are public or private, in comprehensive all-purpose agencies, or in a variety of separate agencies, are among the structural features of a local service system that can have an important effect on who is served.

Finally, statutory and other *legal mandates* have an enormous impact on who is served. In Chapter 2, several statutory landmarks and judicial decisions in the field are described, including the Education for All Handicapped Children Act (PL 94-142) that mandated educational and related services for school-age children. Advocates argue that a similar statutory mandate is required to ensure appropriate early intervention services for preschool children with special needs (Cohen, Semmes, & Guralnick, 1979; Smith, 1984). The priority given to serving severely disabled people that was embodied in the Rehabilitation Act of 1973 is another example of a statutory mandate that has an important effect on who gains access to services (Galvin, 1982). Judicial decisions have had the effect of ensuring that individuals covered by the judicial mandate receive priority in access to developmental services. Similarly, regulations and other legal mandates, statewideness, and comparability in Title XIX (Medicaid), for example, affect who gains access to developmental services.

In sum, a large number of sociodemographic, situational, and environmental factors affect access to services. As certain factors, such as prior institutionalization, become less powerful, there are few, if any, reliable methods for measuring the reciprocal and cumulative impact of other sets of characteristics on need.

CONCLUSION

The growth of community-based developmental services is unquestionably a positive development. However, the increase in the volume and variety of developmental services has brought with it some questions and concerns that are at the core of the field, but have not been adequately addressed or, at least, have been deferred.

There are many more people with severe developmental disabilities living in the community than are now receiving services. In addition to the considerable epidemiologic problems of calculating a prevalence rate for this population, there are several major political dimensions to these statistics. Advocates for previously unserved and underserved disability groups argue that there are exponentially larger numbers of people in need than policy-makers and planners have estimated. Several analysts argue convincingly that the definition of disability must be considered in the context of an individual's familial and programmatic situation. Proposed legislation, such as the Chafee-Florio bill, would broaden definitions of severe developmental disability to encompass many more people in that category. In contrast, proposed changes in Title XIX Medicaid regulations would remove autism from the group of developmental disabilities. The epidemiologic effects of a functional rather than a categorical definition are also unclear. What should be clear is that although there are significant academic and clinical elements to the question of "Who's out there?," there are also important political dimensions to the answer.

The answer to the question of "Who gains access to developmental services?" also has a number of political, economic, and environmental aspects. Increased demand for community-based services is one of the most important elements of this issue. With 10 years of experience with the Education for All Handicapped Children Act, more young people with developmental disabilities have been served by programs to assist them in leading productive adult lives. They and their families expect that a full range of services and supports will be available and accessible for them as adults, and they have become an important political force for expanding the array of services. The desire for access to services in one's own community in contrast to placement in an institution removed from that community will also increase demand. Moreover, the episodic and intermittent services that do not entail lifelong or long-term programming makes them more attractive to larger numbers of people. Finally, the introduction of such new services as family supports and crisis intervention increases the constituencies of developmental services and the demand. Thus, another major dimension to the question of who gains access to services is the increase in their availability. The greater their availability, the greater the demand.

A variety of structural features of the service system also have an important impact on who is served. The creation of ICFs/MR and other more intensive service modalities to serve people being deinstitutionalized not only involves a preference for those people but also establishes a bias toward serving similarly disabled persons from the community or forces inappropriate services on people who do not need an intensive level of care. Thus, the type of services, the auspice of the provider, the degree of service integration among agencies, and other structural features of programs have important effects on who is served.

The service system and environmental factors establish structural parameters that have a pervasive and long-term impact on who is served, and their collective impact is only now emerging as a concern for advocates and policy-makers. At the level of individual demands there are a wide variety of sociodemographic and situational characteristics that have an impact on need for and use of developmental services. Yet, their reciprocal and collective effects are not well understood. Moreover, there is little knowledge about how program, agency, and service system managers use these factors to make decisions about who receives services. On one level, that decision involves the establishment of eligibility criteria and methods to assess the multiple characteristics of individuals seeking services. On another level, the fundamental question of equity of access to services is involved.

It is difficult to consider the question of equity in the context of admission to an institution. However, as community-based developmental services become more available and desirable, that issue becomes more prominent. There is a presumption of equity of access to public services: access that is not necessarily uniform but is based on need and other explicit and agreed-upon criteria. One important aspect of the establishment of community-based services is the shift from public to private provision of services. In most instances, private voluntary agencies have criteria for admission that are similar to publicly operated agencies. However, there are differences, which include preference for less-disabled clients, religious and cultural identification, and suggestions that parents' contribution of time, effort, and money to an agency may influence admission to its programs. With private proprietary agencies, the ability to pay may be a significant factor in determining access to services. For the most part, these questions have not been explicitly and adequately addressed by policy-makers and other significant actors. However, as community-based services grow and are operated by a mix of state government, local government, private voluntary, and private proprietary providers, and as that mix varies across locales, the issue of equity of access will become more prominent and problematic.

The question of who receives services obviously involves deciding who among many individuals seeking access to an insufficient number of services will be served. Who is out there and potentially a seeker of services, what are the characteristics of these individuals that affect their need for and use of services, how does the environment and structure of the service system affect demand and access, who will decide, on what basis; and through what mechanisms are some of the questions that do not now have adequate answers.

5

The Organization of Community-Based Developmental Services

THROUGHOUT THIS BOOK A VARIETY OF POLITICAL, ECONOMIC, AND SO-ciodemographic factors that affect the availability and accessibility of community-based developmental services are examined. Chapter 4 describes how various sociodemographic characteristics of people with developmental disabilities affect their ability to gain access to the services available in a community. This chapter describes how the ways in which those services are organized affect the ability of disabled people to gain access to them.

The term "organization of services" refers to a variety of concerns. One important issue is the types of agencies that provide developmental services: whether they primarily or exclusively serve developmentally disabled people; their size; the number and types of programs they operate; and their auspice, such as governmental, voluntary, or proprietary. Another issue is the ways in which services are delivered; for example, where they are delivered, whether they are delivered alone or in conjunction with other services, and whether they are purchased or provided in-kind. These and similar characteristics of the organization of developmental services affect the accessibility of these services.

One basic premise of this book is that community-based services are significantly different from institutional care. Deinstitutionalization, at least at the outset, has often entailed moving people from large institutions to disaggregated, mini-institutions closer to population centers or nearer their families' homes. For many people, particularly those with mental illness, transinstitutionalization has taken place as they have moved from state hospitals to shelters for the homeless, jails, single-room occupancy hotels, and other community-based institutions. Traditional models of day and residential services that either have been moved to the community context or have grown rapidly as a result of deinstitutionalization have also begun to undergo positive, substantial changes as a result of political, economic, and sociodemographic forces at work in the community. Moreover, new models of developmental services, possible only in a community context, have emerged. In general, developmental services are undergoing important changes in the ways in which they are organized, and this has a crucial impact on how people with developmental disabilities gain access to them.

This chapter is structured around these dimensions of the organization of developmental services. First, the impact of political and economic factors on traditional models of developmental services in the community is discussed. However, because changes in vocational programs and other traditional services have already received considerable attention, they are not re-examined at length here. The focus is largely on some important new models of service and the political and economic ramifications of their emergence.

CHANGES IN TRADITIONAL MODELS OF SERVICES

Vocational Services in the Community

No area has drawn as much attention in the developmental disabilities field or has had as much of an impact on the organization of community-based services as vocational programs. Several recent analyses of employment options for people with developmental disabilities provide excellent analyses of innovative developments in the vocational area (Kiernan & Ciborowski, 1985; Kiernan & Stark, 1986; National Association of Rehabilitation Facilities, 1985; Wehman, 1981).

These innovations in employment for people with developmental disabilities have come about as a result of a variety of political and economic factors. Clearly, the special educational and related services mandated by PL 94-142 have had an enormous impact. Young people with developmental disabilities have not only acquired skills through these services, but, more important, through the experience with their peers without disabilities they have acquired enhanced expectations about entering the adult world of work. Traditional segregated day programs are less and less appropriate for the members of the PL 94-142 generation. These forces have led to important statutory and programmatic initiatives. The Developmental Disabilities Act of 1984 (PL 98-527), for example, included employment-related activities as a priority service. That act defined supported employment as:

> paid employment which (a) is for persons with developmental disabilities for whom competitive employment at or above the minimum wage is unlikely and who, because of their disabilities, need intensive on-going support to perform in a work setting; (b) is conducted in a variety of settings, particularly work sites in which persons without disabilities are employed; and (c) is supported by an activity needed to sustain paid work by persons with disabilities, including supervision, training, and transportation.

The Office of Special Education and Rehabilitative Services has funded supported employment initiatives in several states. In 1981 changes in the Social Security Act (Sections 1619 a and 1619b) reduced, on a time-limited basis, some of the disincentives that existed between receipt of SSI and employment (Conley et al., 1986). These political and economic factors, coupled with a greater appreciation of the capacities for independence of people with developmental disabilities, have resulted in the development of several new models of vocational programs.

The success of innovative vocational programs depends to a large extent on a greater emphasis on preparing for transition to work from schools (Bangser, 1985; Kerachsky et al., 1985; Wehman, Kregel, Barcus, & Schalock, 1986), the provision of additional transitional employment services, and such comprehensive approaches to employment as the Pathways Model (Kiernan & Stark, 1986). The new vocational programs themselves have taken a variety of forms. Some introduce greater flexibility and diversity of programs into traditional rehabilitation facilities, such as hiring more nondisabled employees in workshops and having disabled employees outside the workshop in mobile work crews or in industry-integrated sites (Campbell, 1985). In the job coach model, an individual is placed in competitive employment with a job coach who gradually fades out of supervision as the person becomes more proficient and self-sufficient (Wehman, 1981). A number of other vocational programs and employment options have emerged in recent years, and all of these have shown that people with developmental disabilities can and do participate in the work force to a much greater extent than might be expected from traditional models (Conley, 1973).

The impact of these changes has been felt within a relatively short period of time. One recent survey showed a more than 40 percent increase in the number of adults with developmental disabilities being placed in competitive employment (Kiernan & Ciborowski, 1985). Other studies have also shown very positive results for disabled individuals participating in innovative vocational programs (Shestakofsky, Van Gelder, & Kiernan, 1986; Wehman & Kregel, 1985). The primary focus of these studies has naturally been on the success of individuals in securing and retaining employment.

The continued success of these vocational programs for more people with more severe disabilities will have an important impact on the organization of services for people with developmental disabilities. The rehabilitation agency will become more of the facilitator of employment than the employer. Conversely, for a larger proportion of people with developmental disabilities, employment will increasingly separate them from the segregated, congregate way of life of adult developmental day services.

As discussed in Chapter 3, these new vocational services are having an impact on traditional sheltered workshops. Private agencies do have substantial investments in buildings and equipment in traditional sheltered workshop configurations. Interviews with several agency directors and association executives clearly revealed their concern that public funding for employment programs was increasingly devoted to the innovative types of programs noted above and that both the perceived diminution in funding and the diversion of potential clients to more independent vocational settings would jeopardize the stability of their facilities and agencies. Although the individual with a developmental disability may achieve greater independence through work, that person may still require or desire a group home of some type, need such other support services as transportation or counseling, and may require assistance in negotiating the peculiar linkages between earnings and SSI and SSDI. Many of those services and supports have been provided within or as a result of enrollment in traditional workshop programs (Castellani et al., 1986). The increasing independence of many more persons through employment must be examined for its effects on the organization of these support services and resources.

Residential Programs

Although many people with developmental disabilities who had previously lived in large institutions now live with their families or in other independent settings, the great majority of these individuals moved to community-based congregate care settings (Hill, Lakin, & Bruininks, 1984). Many of these individuals require the relatively structured services of an ICF/MR Program. Many persons who had never been institutionalized have also been placed in community-based ICFs/MR and other structured community residences. Nonetheless, there is a need to develop more residential alternatives for people with developmental disabilities, especially types of housing with less intensive staffing and support (Lakin et al., 1986). Such options as supervised or supported apartments in which one or a small number of persons with developmental disabilities can live with minimal or even occasional assistance are becoming increasingly important.

These new residential programs, which themselves are new ways of organizing community services, have a broader effect on agencies that provide services to people with developmental disabilities and on the overall organization of services in a community.

Medical Services

Large institutions, as well as community-based ICFs/MR, are heavily medicalized environments. Traditional staffing patterns in institutions and the ICF/MR standards result in a very high ratio of physician and nursing staff to the individuals with developmental disabilities. Yet, the lack of available and accessible medical services in communities has been noted as a factor in (re)institutionalization (Gollay et al., 1978; Scheerenberger, 1975).

Within the past few years a number of major changes have occurred in the health care field that will affect the availability and accessibility of medical services for people with developmental disabilities. First, the supply of both hospital beds and physicians has gone from shortage to glut within the past few years. As a result, people with developmental disabilities, together with others who may possess characteristics that did not make them attractive patients, are much more likely to find hospital and physician services more available and accessible. Second, major changes are occurring in the organization of medical services that are likely to increase their accessibility to people with developmental disabilities (Buehler, Menolascino, & Stark, 1986). The rapid expansion in enrollment in such prepaid medical services as health maintenance organizations (HMOs) and the growing use of preferred provider organizations (PPOs) give greater economic leverage to public and private agencies to negotiate either enrollment in HMOs or contracts with PPOs for their clientele. In contrast to the disaggregation of vocational and residential services, medical services for people with developmental disabilities in communities are likely to become more structured through interorganizational arrangements.

Summary

This brief review of changes in vocational, residential, and medical services indicates that traditional models of services are undergoing major changes in the community context. Despite the more corporate character of medical care, most of these changes point toward an increasing diversity in the ways in which services are organized. There also is a movement toward more individualized and less congregate organization of services, especially in the vocational and residential areas. These changes are important and have important effects on other areas of service as well.

NEW MODELS OF COMMUNITY SERVICES: FAMILY SUPPORTS

Family support services have become one of the fastest growing and prominent new models of service in the community. These services are especially important because their implementation has begun to demonstrate that community-based services are qualitatively different from institutional models that have been disaggregated and moved closer to population centers. The way in which these services evolved, the objectives they are expected to achieve, the range of services provided under their framework, the eligibility criteria for access, how they are delivered, and the financing of these services are influenced by political, economic, and sociodemographic factors that are not only important to the development of these services but are also having a significant impact on the availability and accessibility of the entire range of community-based services. Although family support services are regarded as an important and generally positive element of the development of community-based services, the tensions that have developed around the issues noted above raise some fundamental questions about the overall structure of community-based services.

Historical Background

Support services are those services, in addition to core residential and habilitative services, that developmentally disabled people require for normal community life (Scheerenberger, 1975). The development of these family support services has come with the large-scale deinstitutionalization of developmentally disabled people within the past 10 to 15 years. A rather wide range of services are typically included in the framework, such as transportation, recreation, information and referral, respite, diagnosis and evaluation, and parent training. It was generally assumed that these services should be and would be available and accessible to people with developmental disabilities who had moved from large institutions to community-based residences. However, several studies of deinstitutionalized individuals demonstrated that these "generic" services were often not available in communities or, if available, were not accessible to people with developmental disabilities. Gaps in these key services were shown to be related to reinstitutionalization and lack of success in community living (Bachrach, 1981; Braddock, 1981; Gollay et al., 1978; Intagliata et al., 1980).

The support services that were available and accessible to those disabled persons who had been deinstitutionalized were often provided as adjuncts to those persons' day programs (e.g., sheltered workshops or clinics) (New York State Office of Mental Retardation and Developmental Disabilities, 1983). Several states recognized the need in this area and began to generate more fully developed arrays of such support services (Bates, 1983; NASMRPD, 1979).

The literature pays virtually no specific attention to the general definition of family support services. The few studies in this area that deal with definitional issues focus largely on taxonomies of these services: direct and supportive (Bruininks, 1979); hard services, process skills, and counseling skills (Kadushin, 1980; Moroney, 1981); and habilitative family care and ordinary family care (Horejsi, 1979). There is no well-articulated definition of family support services, but rather an apparent consensus around loosely linked concepts and a broad range of services that have become known as family support services. Moreover, an examination of the availability and accessibility of family support services in New York State showed that they were often subsumed in other services and are only identified and defined as family support services because of arbitrary analytic frameworks (New York State Office of Mental Retardation and Developmental Disabilities, 1983).

The recent history of the development of these services also indicates the definitional ambiguity. As was pointed out earlier, the need for support services first became apparent as their absence was shown to be related to reinstitutionalization and lack of success in community living (Bachrach, 1981; Braddock, 1981; Gollay et al., 1978; Intagliata et al., 1980). These previously institutionalized individuals were the primary focus in the development of these services, although the overwhelming majority of people with developmental disabilities live at home with their families and often need the same type of services. To a large degree, support services to this latter group were developed subsequent to and with less resources than were those for the former group. Thus, the services that have become widely known as *family* support services were initially and largely developed as *placement* support services. This historical perspective on defining family support services continues to be very important for their future development because it permeates the policy questions of who are the intended recipients of family support services and what objectives are expected to be achieved through their provision.

Several surveys of the implementation of family support services programs show that virtually the entire range of therapeutic and ancillary services are being provided under this umbrella (Agosta, Bradley, Jennings, Feinberg, & Gettings, 1984; Bates, 1983; NASMRPD, 1979). The historical and conceptual ambiguity surrounding the development of these services is reflected in considerable variation in what states see as family support services. That is, there seems to be a lack of consensus as to what is or is not a family support service or what services are to be included in a family support services program. Thus, the question of what options should be pursued seems to rest, in the first instance, on what is politically and fiscally prudent in attempting to enhance the availability of these services.

The widespread attention given to family support services by professionals and advocates, the increased number of states instituting programs in the area, and the increase in the number of services provided under this framework by states with family support services programs suggest an inclusive strategy. This may be very attractive in the short-term. However, in the long run, this approach carries with it the risk of encompassing such a broad array of services that political support for it will be dissipated. This loss of political support may occur because of the inability to define clearly what is needed or because the costs of the apparently open-ended list of services desired will soon frighten legislators and others who will be called upon to fund these programs.

Eligibility for Family Support Services

The question of whom should be the recipients of family support services is a key issue in this area, and as with the others, it is complex and problematic. It entails both a strategic issue encompassing the overall focus of family support services and the more practical, but nettlesome, issues of how specific eligibility determinations are to be made. Both issues have important political dimensions.

To a large degree, these issues are linked to the basic goals expressed for family support services: 1) strengthening the family structure to enhance the quality of care that families provide to a developmentally disabled member and 2) preventing out-of-home placement (Agosta et al., 1984). A close examination of these goals with respect to eligibility for family support services reveals a major problem. That is, choosing to strengthen families seems to argue for a very broad definition of whom should be the recipient of these services. Indeed, Moroney (1981) proposes a family subsidy that would entail the universal provision of benefits to families caring for a developmentally disabled family member at home. However, at a time when social welfare entitlements are being reconsidered, the use of an entitlement strategy would not seem to be politically feasible.

Another problem with a more universal approach toward strengthening families caring for a developmentally disabled member is the definition of developmental disability. The inclusion of autism, neurological impairment, and learning disability in the definition of developmental disability adds significant problems in ascertaining the number of individuals and families that might become eligible under that broader framework. Advocates for these groups of disabled people have often argued that their numbers are substantially larger than estimates used by government agencies. Moreover, these advocates have been especially vociferous in demanding services for what are believed to be unserved and underserved populations who typically live at home or in other independent community settings. This is especially important because advocates for these disability groups view family support services as a vehicle for access into the developmental services system and a mechanism for overall expansion of services (Castellani & Puccio, 1984).

Finally, this aspect of the eligibility issue raises concerns about competition for services among disability groups. It has been shown that access to family support services is highly dependent on enrollment in regular and routine day programs, which are more typically used by people with mental retardation (Castellani et al., 1986). The advocates and providers of services for mentally retarded persons have been publicly supportive of family support services for a range of disability groups. Informally, they have been more cautious because they are aware that, in an era of continuing scarcity of resources, additional services for other disability groups may result in less services for those currently being served. Thus, a general entitlement approach may create competition between those currently enrolled in programs, and thereby receiving family support services as well, and those other groups of developmentally disabled persons who have been outside the service system and who desire new services, such as family support services.

Another aspect of the problem of a universal approach to eligibility implied in the goal of strengthening families concerns the potential shifting of clients from generic to specialized services. Many people with developmental disabilities, particularly those with autism, learning disabilities, cerebral palsy, and other neurological impairments, are currently receiving services from social service, health, mental health, and rehabilitation service providers. The expansion of services to those living at home, particularly those people with low-incidence disorders, creates the possibility that clients and families currently served by other systems may move into the developmental disabilities service system through the vehicle of family support services. This move may be needed and appropriate. However, the political and administrative energy needed to extend services to the unserved and underserved may be dissipated if trading already served clients among service domains results.

Financing these family services looms as a central concern of the broad approach to eligibility. Clearly, providing a modicum of services to all families to strengthen their capacity to care for a member with a developmental disability can be very costly. A basic question is whether few services are to be provided to virtually all families in this category or whether more services are to be provided to those most in need.

Delivery of Family Support Services

One of the most important concerns in the delivery of services is the *level of government* best suited to manage these services. There are significant differences between managing a large and bureaucratically oriented system of institutions and overseeing a more personalized and individualized program of family support services. In some ways, even community residences and ICFs/MR are imposed on communities, and federal and state regulatory structures tend to ensure uniformity in those service models. Family support services, however, are linked more intimately to the communities in which they operate than other residential and day programs. The diversity of communities suggests that the management structure be flexible. The relatively uniform management models that were designed to operate very similar institutions across a state cannot be expected to function well in various community settings.

Another concern is the extent to which family support services are intended to conform to or compensate for *community conditions*. At stake here is a basic question of equity within and among locales. Much more needs to be known about the environment within which family support services programs operate. Clearly, family support services are related to such community resources as the availability and accessibility of public transportation, recreational facilities, medical, dental, and other professional services, and these services and resources vary greatly by locale. In one respect, local management of family support services can best take into account local needs and resources. Yet, the intimate link between family support services and often widely varying community resources raises the question of whether and to what extent family support services should be provided in amount and type to equalize the differences in availability and accessibility that are likely to result. Clearly, institutional models, especially those supported in part through Medicaid funding, are operated in large part on the principles of "statewideness" and equal access. Placement support services, as pointed out earlier, were in many instances initially built around community residences for deinstitutionalized persons and served as models for family support services for individuals who had never resided in an institution. They created a strong precedent for equalizing the availability and accessibility of family support services across local governments to compensate for comparative deficits in resources and services.

The *relationship between the public and private sectors,* including voluntary and proprietary agencies, is another concern that must be addressed in the delivery of family support services. Many states have a widely varying array of state government, local government, and private agencies involved in the management and delivery of community-based services. The dominance of one or another sector in various locales is a function of historical, political, economic, and other factors that may confound rational program design, but are nonetheless powerful in conditioning the shape of programs. Depending upon the auspice of the provider, management and delivery of family support services may result in different outcomes.

Private proprietary management and ownership of acute and long-term care health facilities have provided examples of economies of scale and models of efficiency that may merit consideration for the management of at least some family support services for developmentally disabled people (Zuckerman, 1983). An obvious concern, however, is accessibility to services by clients and families who may present complex, unusual, and troublesome problems that make them commercially unattractive. Private voluntary agencies may also be unwilling to serve these clients. Moreover, many private voluntary agencies have traditional disability orientations and religious, ethnic, racial, and geographical identifications or affiliations that limit accessibility to many families in need of support services.

State government has been the provider of last resort and might be expected to provide a management structure ensuring the greatest degree of availability and accessibility (NYS OMRDD, 1983). However, state government–operated services tend to be the most expensive, and their institutional bias and historical perspective may inhibit delivery of family support services to unserved and underserved populations (Commission on Quality of Care for the Mentally Disabled [NYS], 1984).

The use of *public nonprofit agencies* established for the purpose of managing the delivery of family support services is another structural option. A key issue is the degree of authority that type of agency might exercise over other governmental agencies in coordinating and gaining access to services for its clientele.

A range of structural possibilities are suggested here. One model need not be selected to the exclusion of others across an entire state, and several models could function conjointly or collaboratively. Family support services represent a substantially distinct type of service, and it should not be assumed that management models derived from institutional perspectives or even community residential and day program services can be appropriately or easily adapted for family support services.

The degree to which *families are empowered* to exercise choice in the amount, type, source, and use of family support services seems to be emerging as one of the most central and politically sensitive issues affecting the delivery of family support services. The basic question concerns the structure of services and the mechanisms that families can use to gain access to those services.

Many states began support services programs when it became apparent that people who had been placed out of institutions were returning or having problems because the so-called generic services that were expected to be available were not. It has often been only secondarily that states have provided support services to families as spinoffs of placement support services or in belated recognition of the needs of families caring for a developmentally disabled member at home. Thus, the progression has been first to ensure that those services that had been available in institutions were provided to individuals placed in the community and then to attempt to make those services available to people living at home with their families. In many instances, these family support services are provided as direct service adjuncts to core residential and day programs (Castellani et al., 1986).

The increasing demand for and use of family support services have raised several problems and concerns with the direct provision of services model. With increasing experience, it is becoming clearer that families are radically different from institutions, even those that are community-based. The structure of service delivery is primarily institutional, and the problems and opportunities that families present seem to confound or be confounded by that structure.

The family home is often the setting where family support services are provided. In many instances, the family is the provider of services. The family is also the consumer of services, and these roles often occur at the same time. Government regulations, policies, guidelines, and funding formulas do not typically or easily deal with the somewhat simultaneous overlap of roles that occur in providing family support services.

One response to these problems has been to increase the array of services available in family support programs. However, this still results in a product-driven system. That is, families' choices are limited to the services made available by the state or agencies contracted to provide family support services.

Another response to these concerns is the use of cash subsidies and/or vouchers by an increasing number of family support services programs. Cash subsidies and vouchers, although limited in amount and occasionally to specific types of services, are an important alternative to direct provision of services. They increase the discretionary power of the family, and in light of the complexity of dealing with the family as provider and consumer, the simplicity of cash subsidy approaches may be more attractive to governments. It does seem, nevertheless, that the same political energy that is resulting in demand for more family support services is also resulting in greater demands for approaches and mechanisms that empower the family. This suggests that family support services represent an increasingly significant departure in the way in which services are provided to people with developmental disabilities and their families and may ultimately have a similar effect on the entire range of community-based services.

Financing Family Support Services

The financing of family support services is the last major dimension that has important ramifications for the organization of community-based services. Although it has been very difficult to identify the funding sources of family support services in the organizational contexts in which they are often provided (Castellani et al., 1986), it is nonetheless clear that states are now the primary source of funding for family support services (Braddock, Hemp, & Howes, 1985c). However, the Home and Community Care Waiver and the proposed Community and Family Living Amendments will most likely greatly expand federal funding of these services. Family support services are peculiarly local in nature, and yet the role of local government in this area is uncertain. It is generally assumed that local governments that depend in large measure on property and sales taxes for revenue have neither the capacity nor willingness to fund family support services programs themselves. However, some core family support services, such as transportation and recreation, are services typically provided by local governments. Voluntary agencies that provide substantial amounts of such services as respite, counseling, and information and referral also rely in part on funding from local government sources. Moreover, school districts, either as independent local entities or as components of municipal governments, are being pressured to provide more family support services as adjuncts to special education services mandated by PL 94-142. Thus, although the role of local government in funding family support services has not been the subject of much discussion, closer attention must be paid to the problems and opportunities of financing at this level of government.

Some attention has been paid to private sources of funding for family support services (Agosta et al., 1984), particularly through inclusion of these services either in privately purchased or employer-provided health insurance programs. The potentially large and usually long-term costs associated with services (including family support services) for persons with developmental disabilities tend either to confound basic insurance principles or prove to be prohibitively expensive (Bishop, 1981; Kane & Kane, 1978). Proposals for publicly financed national childhood disability insurance (Gliedman & Roth, 1980) have not generated as much interest as direct government provided or funded services programs. Generally, the focus of attention for funding family support services has been on public rather than private sources.

Summary

Family support services are an important new model of community-based services, and their implementation has far-reaching implications for the entire range of community-based developmental services. The evolution of these services from placement support services has brought into sharper relief the distinction between services moved from institutions to the community and community-based services. The rationale for their establishment—preventing institutionalization and strengthening families—has also pointed out the need to establish more carefully a rationale for community-based services that is independent of the linkage to institutionalization.

Family support services are particularly important in providing access to a fairly wide range of therapeutic and supportive services to families whose members have never been institutionalized. Although that broad and ambiguous definition of these services may be politically troublesome, family support services are an important vehicle for access to developmental services for groups of disabled individuals who have typically been unserved or underserved. Broad and ambiguous eligibility criteria also raise concerns about the degree to which family support services are a mechanism of a more general family policy that extends beyond the traditional focus of developmental services.

The ways in which family support services have been delivered, particularly the use of cash subsidies and vouchers, have had an important impact on their availability and accessibility. First, these mechanisms tend to empower families in dealing with traditional service organizations in this area, and they provide important precedents for a wider use of such mechanisms in other areas of developmental services. Second, family support services are one important focus of attempts to restructure the federal funding of developmental services. Their development has been in many respects the counterpoint of proposals to defund institutional models of care. In general, family support services are a very important component of community-based developmental services, and their implementation is having a significant impact on the ways in which community-based services are organized.

OTHER NEW MODELS OF COMMUNITY SERVICES

Home Care

Home care is closely related to family support services, although the services are focused more on meeting the needs of the disabled client outside institutional settings than on the needs of families (Perlman & Giele, 1983; Seidl, Applebaum, Austin, & Mahoney, 1983). Nonetheless, the extensive use of these services, particularly for elderly individuals, has encouraged analysts, advocates, and policy-makers to urge the possible broader application for individuals with developmental disabilities (New York City Human Resources Administration, 1984; Perlman, 1985). Despite a number of reports of the positive impact of home care (Birnbaum, Burke, Swearingen, & Dunlop, 1984), there are also indications that home care presents problems in the organization and coordination of services.

Brecher and Knickman (1985) argue, "A number of studies and reports reveal that expanded provision of home care, while having much merit, does not substantially reduce institutionalization, generates added costs, and sometimes leads families to reduce the time they spend caring for elderly relatives" (p. 245). Moreover, their review of several home care experiments indicated that new funds were absorbed by additional clients. In general, the implementation of home care provides important experience with service models, reimbursement systems, and service coordination that may be important as a way of organizing and providing services for people with developmental disabilities. The experience also indicates that home care is not the "silver bullet" that it was expected to be.

Crisis Intervention Services

As the focus of developmental services turns increasingly toward the needs of disabled people in the community, it is important to keep in mind that the great majority of these individuals do not live in con- gregate care or supportive residential facilities or attend highly structured day programs. Nevertheless, the developmentally dis- abled people who live and work outside those settings may be as disabled as many who do participate in them (Kiernan & Bruininks, 1986). They may also face long-term problems or encounter more acute difficulties that may threaten their well-being, cause them to lose their jobs or housing, and may lead them to be placed in more restrictive settings: in developmental services, mental health facili- ties, or jail. A question that has emerged is the extent to which services intended to meet the intermittent, episodic, or crisis needs of developmentally disabled people not in congregate care or family settings should be a component of community-based developmental services or left to other human service providers.

Crisis intervention services have been developed in New York State, for example, as response to specific situations or problems faced by people with developmental disabilities that threaten their well-being and place them in jeopardy of institutionalization, but do not entail the long-term relationships usually associated with case management services (Commission on Quality of Care, 1984b). The services may include counseling, advocacy, and other short-term interventions. Most of these services are directed to people living in family care homes with their own families or in other group homes. However, some services are provided to developmentally disabled people who live on their own and do not receive other routine devel- opmental services. The situations requiring attention by community service staff of state or contract developmental service agencies usu- ally involve loss of a job or housing, maladaptive behavior, transpor- tation problems, or other difficulties of this type. However, people with developmental disabilities are sometimes also involved in more serious problems, such as criminal assault, larceny, homicide, and other behaviors that involve the police and the courts. These more serious problems, especially when they are manifested by developmentally disabled people who do not participate in residential and day services, raise the question of the extent to which crisis intervention services should be components of community-based developmental services or should be parts of other human service systems, including criminal justice.

The implementation of all types of community-based programs has made these developmental services more visible. The creation of such other-than-total care models as family support services also make developmental services more accessible. This accessibility, in combination with the absence of clear-cut eligibility criteria and the little, if any, information about who may need or demand these services, has some important implications. On the one hand there is some sentiment that community-based developmental services should not extend to providing crisis intervention services to people with developmental disabilities, however severe, who have never been institutionalized or are not now in routine day or residential services or who are involved in criminal or seriously antisocial behavior. On the other hand, much of the thrust to implement community-based services comes from advocates who argue that it is the needs of people with disabilities that should determine the services they get, rather than prior institutionalization, place of residence, enrollment in day programs, or other similar factors (Commission on Quality of Care, 1984b). This pull and push between resource allocators and advocates is one aspect of the situation that will define the extent of crisis intervention services. However, another important concern is the response of other human services agencies, including the criminal justice system, to crisis intervention services. Currently, there are overcrowded jails, clogged court calendars, mental health facilities with neither the capacity nor inclination to deal with developmentally disabled people, and other overloaded service areas that might otherwise handle crises. Too, many other human services agencies are only recently discovering that many of their clients are having problems because they have a developmental disability. It is very likely that crisis intervention services will increasingly become vehicles for these other agencies to transfer developmentally disabled people with a variety of problems to the developmental service system.

Crisis intervention services are highlighted because they are a relatively new model of service. More importantly, they illustrate the fact that implementation of a new model of service creates important effects in a broader range of human services. Some of those effects may be unknown or unintended. Nonetheless, they do have significant consequences for the organization of services for people with developmental disabilities.

Early Intervention Services

One of the most troublesome areas in community-based services is the organization of services for developmentally disabled children from their birth to the time they receive full educational and related services. The passage of PL 94-142 was a major landmark in the field of community-based services for people with developmental disabilities. Although there have been substantial problems achieving full implementation of the mandates of that act, its basic policy objectives—to secure for disabled children the educational services they require to achieve their full potential—is clear. Moreover, these children are served within the organization of schools until the age of 22, which despite a variety of problems, involves rather clear-cut models of services, eligibility criteria, funding mechanisms, and linkages to other service systems.

It is generally agreed that early intervention services for children with handicapping conditions, especially those with developmental delays, should begin as soon as possible after birth (Dunst, 1985; Dunst & Rheingrover, 1981; Tjossem, 1976). However, there are no consistent clear-cut legal mandates or sets of policy objectives that guide the delivery of services for disabled children until they are enrolled in formal educational services. As a result, there is a corresponding absence of a comprehensive and cohesive framework for the organization of early intervention services.

Questions to be resolved about the organization of services for young children include, among others, the service domain into which early intervention services fall (health, education, social services, MR/DD), the type of organizations that provide those services, the various service models, eligibility criteria for access to services, and funding. These issues are all of significance to the availability and accessibility of these (and all other) community-based developmental services. They are particularly interesting because, in the absence of clear legal mandates, policy guidelines, and the hegemony of any one service domain, the variety of political and economic factors affecting their availability and accessibility can be more readily seen.

When considering early intervention services for very young children with developmental disabilities, a question that is often raised is "whose children are these?" What should be obvious is that services, eligibility, funding, and a variety of other crucial aspects of care are substantially different across the major service domains that might come into play—medical, educational, and social welfare.

When the presence of a severe developmental disability, especially one requiring medical-surgical services, is evident at birth, the disabled child falls immediately in the medical domain. In those cases, access to services is largely a function of birth with a disability, and services are typically provided in the hospital-clinic environment. The hospital-clinic may also be the organizational framework for a broader range of ancillary and support services to the child and the family. Funding for services, however, can be a serious problem for the family as it not only faces large expenses but also the vagaries of private insurance reimbursement, out-of-pocket expenditures, and Medicaid eligibility (Kakalik et al., 1981). Reforms, such as Model 50 waivers that fund home care for disabled children at risk of hospitalization, have begun to address some of those funding problems. It is still the case, however, that access to services and reimbursement for their cost in the medical domain remain almost inextricably linked to prior and/or risk of hospitalization.

Once a child leaves the hospital, the child and family face an extremely complex environment of services should a developmental delay become apparent or be suspected, and there are several distinct service domains, organizations, and models for early intervention. However, the first problem is obtaining those services. Identification of a developmental delay may be very difficult, and even when families have a pediatrician or family practitioner, there are ample indications that primary care physicians very often do not recognize developmental delays, do not readily refer families to developmental specialists, and are often unaware of specialized developmental services in their communities (Blacher, 1984). Very often developmental disabilities go undetected at least until the children enter school.

For those developmentally disabled children who do receive early intervention services, the path to those services may be difficult, and there are several distinct directions that may be taken. First, many states have developed specific mechanisms to identify children with handicaps, including developmental disabilities, and to refer them to diagnostic, evaluation, and early intervention services. In New York and other states for example, Early Childhood Direction Centers have been established under the aegis of the state education department to provide regional outreach, identification, and referral of these children to services and to promote public and professional awareness of handicapping conditions (Zeller, 1980). An Infant Health Assessment Program has also been established in New York with Maternal and Childhood Block grant funding to follow up children whose birth characteristics—low birth weight, young maternal age, prematurity—put them at risk of a handicapping condition. The SSI/Disabled Children's Program, the Child Health Assessment Program, and various child-find services are other mechanisms for identification, outreach, and, in some cases, funding for early intervention services for disabled children. No program, however, is focused specifically on developmental disabilities, and each one's similar objectives and separate organizations indicate the compartmentalized approach in this area as each service domain establishes its own identification and referral capacity.

In addition, access to early intervention services is not dependent on referral through any of the above mechanisms, and one review showed a variety of direct and indirect pathways (Bird, 1984c). In many respects coordination of access to early intervention services is thwarted by the existence of a myriad of provider organizations operating under the various service domains—medical, social welfare, educational—as well as traditional developmental services. An analysis of early intervention services in New York State identified the following types of providers: hospital-based clinics; free-standing clinics; independent providers of early intervention services; and services linked to traditional developmental service providers, such as ARCs, Boards of Cooperative Educational Services (intermediate schools), and a variety of private professional practitioners (Reif, 1985).

In New York State the plethora of early intervention and service providers is related to the various funding sources for these services. In addition to Medicaid, private insurance, or out-of-pocket expenditures, a substantial proportion of early intervention services are ordered on the basis of parent petitions to county family courts, and the costs, which are largely set by the providers, are shared by the county and state government on a 50-50 basis. In the absence of a legal framework, clear policy objectives, local or state regulations, funding guidelines, or oversight mechanisms, the provision of early intervention services in this manner has resulted in an exponential escalation of costs. Over the past several years, total costs for services provided in this manner to approximately 13,000 children annually grew from about $11 million in 1977–1978 to almost $200 million in 1986–1987 (Legislative Commission on Expenditure Review, 1984). Despite the relatively large amounts of funds expended for early intervention services, recent evaluations of these services by local providers and outside experts in the field have pointed to a number of problems of coordination, lack of planning, absence of clear eligibility criteria, and other similar concerns (Albert Einstein College of Medicine, 1986).

There is little evidence by which to measure the outcomes of these services, but the soaring costs, competition for clients, increasing number of providers, and the absence of any significant coordination or oversight in this area illustrate the problems of organization of community-based developmental services. This experience suggests that, although early intervention services may denote specific approaches, therapies, and other hallmarks of professional practice, they do not constitute a cohesive and integrated service domain in the community. Nor does it appear that the myriad of service organizations in the field operate under any coordinated developmental services framework. The absence of a legal framework that establishes clear policy objectives and operational guidelines and a disjointed and compartmentalized array of service systems with various eligibility criteria, funding mechanisms, and types of service providers have led to a complex and confusing system of early intervention services.

Independent Living

Independent living, which is a service model that has emerged within the past several years, represents a distinct but important phenomenon in the organization of community-based services. Several aspects of independent living are significantly different from other community-based models and may have broad implications (Jones, Hannah, Fawcett, Seekins, & Buddle, 1984).

First, independent living is largely designed for people with physical disabilities and cerebral palsy and does not have the traditional focus on mental retardation that typifies services in the developmental services field. In addition to this disability perspective, the movement, as it is termed by its most prominent exponent, Gerben DeJong, has become most active in academic communities, and its constituents are usually well educated. DeJong (1979) not only sees a specific disciplinary orientation in the independent living movement encompassing physical medicine and rehabilitation specialties but also argues that this disciplinary focus entails a conflict with the prevailing rehabilitation paradigm. He further argues that independent living emphasizes consumer sovereignty, benefit rights, self-care, and demedicalization; in addition, there is an explicit anti-parent element in the movement that eschews typical notions of dependency on the part of people with developmental disabilities (DeJong, 1979). Self-directed attendant care, rather than professsional-directed home health services, is seen as the prototype of independent living service (DeJong & Wenker, 1979).

Independent living centers have developed rapidly in the past several years, and this growth suggests some important new directions in the organization of services (New York State Education Department, 1985). In particular, the major emphasis on *independence* is in sharp contrast to the major role that parents have played in advocating for services and actually operating developmental service agencies. The public financing of attendant care is important to independent living. However, the work disincentives created by that point to the need to reconsider the linkages between basic income maintenance and employment. In general, the independent living movement indicates that the broader inclusion of disability groups within the framework of developmental disabilities, the impact of PL 94-142, and new attitudes toward dependency are having important consequences in this area of services. It is very likely that in the future these factors will have broader effects on the organization of community-based services.

CONCLUSION

The major conclusion of this chapter is that the community context of developmental services exerts a powerful influence on the ways those services are organized. Changes in traditional models of developmental services and the emergence of new models influence their future shape.

The continuing existence of large institutions, the process of deinstitutionalization, and the concern for (re)institutionalization of individuals living in communities have been significant factors shaping the ways in which community-based services are organized along that institution-community axis. In some communities the developmental services are predominantly total care and congregate care models of residential and day services, and there are few or no services for people not enrolled in those programs.

Traditional models of vocational, residential, and medical services are undergoing important changes in the community as a result of new political and economic factors. Some of these changes have been brought about directly by statutory and fiscal initiatives from federal and state government, whereas others are results of changes in other service domains. New models of services, such as family supports, crisis intervention, independent living, and early intervention, are emerging, and these are peculiar to the community context and represent significant changes in the organization of services.

The changes in traditional models and the emergence of new models are leading to a greater diversity in the types of service and are being provided by new and different types of service agencies in many cases. Vouchers and cash subsidies for family supports and home care are important new ways of financing services and purchasing services in a broader marketplace. Supported work and family supports, as well as other new types of services, are not provided in congregate care settings and may be largely outside the aegis of traditional provider agencies. Some models of service are used more intermittently and do not entail the long-term client-agency relationship that typifies many traditional service models. They are often provided to a broader and often new clientele who may have never been served by developmental service agencies. In general, these services and new ways of organizing them tend to move the focus of provision toward the individual and away from the service agency. The collective impact of these changes and new models place pressure on traditional service agencies to become more disaggregated.

Deinstitutionalization will occupy the attention of advocates, policy-makers, and providers for some time, and the success of those efforts will lead to a situation where the institutional-community axis will no longer act as the key to the organization of services. People with developmental disabilities who need and seek services in the community are significantly more diverse in the type, frequency, and intensity of their needs than are the relatively stable clients that were served in the early stages of the deinstitutionalization process. The models of service are also becoming more diverse, disaggregated, and less defined by clear-cut organizational boundaries. People with developmental disabilities and the services they use exist and function in an environment in which they, other human services and dependent populations, and the political, economic, and sociodemographic factors in the community interact in a complex interpersonal and interorganizational milieu.

6

Decisions at the
Point of Delivery

THE FOCUS OF THIS CHAPTER IS ON THE WAYS IN WHICH DECISIONS ABOUT developmental services in communities are made and the factors that have a significant impact on those decisions. Its premise is that the shift from large state-operated institutions to smaller facilities in communities entails new decision-making structures, a wide variety of new actors in the policy process, and a new set of problems that are requiring some different and innovative approaches to providing, paying for, managing, and coordinating developmental services.

This chapter begins with a brief review of the history of state and local responsibility for the care of people with mental disabilities that points to the cyclical approaches to responsibility for community-based services. Second, the various dimensions of the local capacity to provide and manage developmental services, including community experience, fiscal capacity, and management capability and willingness to provide these services—are discussed. The next part of the chapter examines intergovernmental relations, problems of decision-making among various governmental bodies within each locale, the question of who decides at the local level, and the important decision-making structures and processes. Finally, the issue of building developmental service systems in the community is discussed, with a focus on problems in coordinating and integrating developmental services and some emerging approaches and mechanisms.

CYCLES OF RESPONSIBILITY FOR CARE

Historically, responsibility for the direct delivery of service for dependent populations, particularly the mentally disabled, has shifted back and forth between state and local government (Deutsch, 1949).

Each shift seems to have left a residual effect on the roles of each level of government (Rothman, 1971).

In colonial America the care of the mentally disabled was haphazard. Under the legacy of the Poor Laws of Elizabethan England, localities were responsible for the care of paupers, vagrants, and the mentally disabled. The levy of a local "poor tax" was earmarked for their care. To reduce this levy, local officials would load a wagon with these individuals and "dump" them off in a neighboring town. Another method for dealing with the dependent population was "boarding out," in which an indigent person was auctioned off to the lowest bidder who would be reimbursed at that price and would receive the services of that person (Derrico, 1982).

Later, increasing urbanization spurred the development of more institutional forms of care, principally the local almshouses that became the depository for a variety of dependent groups. A series of exposés revealed the deplorable conditions in local almshouses and caused a public outcry that led to the establishment of state asylums as a humanitarian reform. The establishment of asylums in the mid-1800s was also an outgrowth of such innovation as Pinel's moral treatment. However, by shortly after the Civil War state asylums had become custodial, and the quality of care was virtually indistinguishable from that found in the almshouse.

In New York, the state took fiscal responsibility for the construction of asylums in the 1840s. The counties were required to reimburse the state at a weekly rate for each resident of the county who received care in the state asylum. In many instances, because it was less expensive for counties to house the mentally disabled in almshouses or to board them out than to pay the costs of state care, a dual system existed for much of the 19th century. During this time, counties lobbied for state assumption of the costs of care, and social reformers argued that a state-operated system would also be more humane and efficient. In 1890, the first comprehensive State Care Act in the country was passed in New York, and all mentally disabled people being cared for in local almshouses were eventually transferred to state care and cost. In its major features, this system remained the same until the development of the concepts of community care for the mentally disabled in the 1950s and 1960s, from which grew the contemporary changes that are outlined in Chapter 1.

This brief historical review glosses over some of the differences in the care provided to the indigent, mentally ill, mentally retarded, and other groups that were involved in the movement between almshouses, asylums, and boarding out. Nonetheless, it points out that the tension between state and local governments over the responsibility of providing services and assuming the costs of care for people with mental disabilities dates back to colonial America. In many respects, the issues and problems that have arisen at the local level regarding the establishment of programs for people with developmental disabilities in community settings are reprises of these historical tensions.

COMMUNITY CAPACITY AND DEVELOPMENTAL SERVICES

In some respects, virtually all human services are local in nature. However, in order for developmental services to be truly community-based and integrated into the fabric of other human services, communities must have the capacity and willingness to assume some major responsibility for supporting and managing those services. This section describes three important elements of this capacity: 1) the general community awareness of developmental disabilities and services; 2) the fiscal capacity and willingness to support developmental services; and 3) the managerial capability to plan, develop, and provide for developmental services.

Experience in Developmental Services

The brief history of the shift in roles between state and local governments in the care of people with mental disabilities indicates that local governments have historically assumed responsibility in this area. Indeed, local governments have traditionally taken primary responsibility in such areas as education, housing, and social services, which are of major significance to people with developmental disabilities. Nonetheless, for most of the 20th century the care of people with developmental disabilities either was provided in large state-operated almshouses or in a few relatively small educational programs run by parent groups or was the total responsibility of parents and other family members. To a large degree, local governments have had very little experience in funding, managing, or providing developmental services.

Although this variable is very difficult to measure, a community's experience with people with developmental disabilities can have an important effect on its development of services. From a negative perspective, the removal of people with developmental disabilities from their homes to large, often remote institutions and their exclusion from schools, hospitals, and other human services resulted in unfamiliarity, fear, hostility, and a variety of other attitudes that presented obstacles to the establishment of service in communities. Those advocates who have presented and defended plans for the creation of community residences often point to the fundamental lack of knowledge about people with developmental disabilities as an enormous barrier to be overcome (Cohen, 1975; Rothman & Rothman, 1984). The confusion and misunderstandings about what are developmental disabilities, the needs of people with those disabilities, and what services and supports are required extend well beyond apprehensive neighbors to the parents of those individuals, government officials, and a wide variety of human service professionals and managers (Bachrach, 1981; Cohen, 1975; Novak, 1980; Runkel, 1985). Large-scale deinstitutionalization, the creation of community programs, and education of handicapped children in public schools have all occurred within the past 10 years, which in terms of human services development is a relatively short period of time. Indeed, one nationally prominent figure in the special education field informally observed that one of the most significant effects of the Education for All Handicapped Children Act was probably the increased sensitivity of nonhandicapped children to people with special needs. Nonetheless, the more specific changes in organization of service and funding rest on an awareness of the existence and needs of people with developmental disabilities and a consensus that communities should provide the services these individuals require.

Fiscal Capacity

Without question, no area of local capacity to provide or play an important role in delivering developmental services is more prominently and vigorously discussed than fiscal capacity. One recent study of the role of local government in mental health and developmental services in 24 states reported that the three essential factors affecting the role of counties were, "funding, funding, and funding" (Jaskulski, 1983a). The fiscal capacity of local governments to maintain existing services has been the topic of substantial analysis in recent years (Accountants for the Public Interest, 1983; Bahl, 1984; Brown, Fossett, & Palmer, 1984; Clark, 1985; Gargan, 1985; Gold, 1983; New York State Governor's Select Commission on the Future of the State-Local Mental Health System, 1984).

Despite the salience of the topic, the findings of these studies regarding the fiscal capacity to support developmental services are somewhat ambiguous. Bahl (1984) points out the complexity of the problem and cautions against generalizations about local governments' fiscal capacity:

> Our complicated local government structure makes it possible for
> some central cities to deteriorate while their suburban neighbors thrive.
> In addition, there is great variation across the country in the distribution
> of taxing powers and expenditure responsibility between levels of gov-
> ernment. (p.5)

There is nonetheless a great deal of anxiety about this fiscal capacity.

Much of the concern about local government finances is generated both by structural factors and some disturbing problems in this
area over the past several years. First, there has been a large overall
expansion in state and local governments in the past 50 years, but
structurally, local governments still remain fiscally vulnerable. State
law usually defines what services must be and may be delivered by
city government and also determines what options are available to
local government for financing those services (Gargan, 1985). Counties are typically limited to generating the bulk of their revenues
through property and sales taxes, and not only are these forms of
revenue rather inflexible but they have been under attack from a
variety of "Proposition 13" and "Proposition 2½" limitations
(Gargan, 1985; Gold, 1983; Jaskulski, 1983b). Moreover, local governments are highly dependent on state and federal aid for substantial portions of their overall revenues (Chubb, 1985). Gold (1983)
notes, "Since aid to local governments is the largest component of
state budgets, state fiscal problems inevitably affect local governments" (p. 1). Gold (1983) also finds that the predominant influence
on state finances in the late 1970s and early 1980s was the weak state
of the national economy. Additionally, both revenue sharing and
direct federal-local government grant programs over the past 10
years have led to the local governments' heightened dependence on
federal aid (Brown et al., 1984; Parker, 1985). Finally, the high inflation and successive recessions of the late 1970s, as well as the antici-
pation of large cuts in federal and, consequently, state aid as a result
of the "New Federalism" of the Reagan administration, created an
overall sense of fiscal vulnerability for local governments (Jaskulski,
1983a; Janovsky, Scallet, & Jaskulski, 1983).

The perception of vulnerability to cutbacks may be as politically
important, if not more so, than the actual cutbacks. Gold (1983)
points out that few of the drastic changes presaged in President
Reagan's "New Federalism" were actually enacted and that the
block grant initiatives have had only a modest effect. Moreover, Gold
concludes, "States have been moving gradually to assume greater
service and financing responsibilities. The state role in financing
elementary and secondary education, welfare, and courts has in-

creased steadily since the 1970s" (p. 2). Nonetheless, the perception of vulnerability persists as counties report mandates without commensurate funding, limited startup costs for programs they are expected to initiate, delayed and inadequate reimbursement for the state's share of those programs, and a variety of other similar problems of local fiscal capacity (Jaskulski, 1983a).

In addition to the reality or perception of a local government's fiscal capacity, a community's willingness to use its resources is another important factor. That willingness is analyzed in the context of tax effort indicators, which are a measure of the extent to which a local government taxes itself to pay for services (Bahl, 1984; Clark, 1985; Nathan & Adams, 1976; Parker, 1985). A number of studies have highlighted the variations among locales in this index of their willingness to use their resources. In the developmental disabilities field, one recent analysis in New York State showed wide variation in the extent to which counties used their tax-levy dollars or relied on voluntary agency contributions to meet their local share of state aid to localities (New York State Office of Mental Retardation and Developmental Disabilities, 1985).

It is difficult to estimate the amount of local financing of developmental services. Braddock and Hemp (1986) estimate that local governments provided approximately $1.6 billion for developmental services in federal fiscal year 1984, which represents about 10.8 percent of the $14.97 billion in federal, state, and local government expenditures in that year. Of that $1.6 billion, Braddock and Hemp (1986) estimate that $1.27 billion (8.5% of the total) was spent on local special education and the remaining $344 million (2.3% of the total) on noneducational developmental services. Although Braddock and his associates have collected a substantial amount of data on federal and state expenditures in the area, their estimate of the nonspecial education expenditures is based on an extrapolation from data from only three states: Virginia, Nebraska, and Wisconsin. Although the data are limited, it is nonetheless apparent that, other than in special education, local governments are not now making substantial contributions to the costs of developmental services.

The overall picture of local government fiscal capacity is somewhat clouded. The perception both of vulnerability and fiscal overburden on the part of local government is well supported in part and in some locales (Clark, 1985). Moreover, those perceptions and their political impact may be more enduring than any feeling of wellbeing brought about by low inflation, a generally improved economy, and the surpluses experienced by many state and local governments in the mid-1980s. In any case, in considering the participation of local government in the establishment of developmental services in communities, the issue of fiscal capacity is likely to be one of the most salient.

Local Government Management Capacity

The capacity and willingness of local governments to finance developmental services are the issues most often raised by local officials. However, the relative fiscal burden on local government is small, and there are indications that states are assuming even greater portions of the costs of human services. Other elements of local capacity are important to the establishment and maintenance of community-based developmental services. Local managerial capacity is especially significant as the number, type, and complexity of developmental services in communities increase. Although local governments may not provide substantial fiscal support for these services, they are increasingly called upon to undertake a variety of managerial responsibilities, and as Gargan (1981) observes, "Local governments in the United States vary in their ability to deal with problems" (p. 648).

Local management capacity is largely determined by capability in three main areas (Study Committee on Policy Management Assistance, 1975):

1. *Policy management,* which typically involves such tasks as needs assessment, planning, establishment of priorities, development of strategies, and mobilization of resources
2. *Resource management,* which entails such functions as personnel, financial, information, and property management.
3. *Program management,* which includes the execution of specific policies by undertaking programs, activities, and services

It has been widely recognized that local governments have serious deficiencies in managerial capacity. Moreover, the specific experience with developmental services is very recent, and most local governments have not had the time to develop much expertise in policy, resource, and financial management of developmental services (Janicki, Castellani, & Norris, 1983).

Management Capacity and Political Willingness

Gargan (1981) argues that "local government capacity should not be viewed exclusively from a management perspective" (p. 7). Important political factors go beyond those management concerns, and they concern such basic interests of local officials as their re-election and avoidance of conflict. Local government political capacity entails interaction among such key dimensions as: 1) *local expectations* about the adequate levels of public service, based on local priorities, traditions, and culture; 2) *local political resources*, including such factors as money, political popularity, neighborhood organizations, and administrative skills; and 3) the *ability to resolve local problems* (Gargan, 1981).

The overwhelming majority of the literature on the establishment of community-based developmental services, as well as the rhetoric of advocates and federal and state policy-makers, is cast in a proactive perspective. The focus of attention is on what programs and services should be implemented, and in this context, what local capacity must be put in place or enhanced in order for local governments to take a greater role. Gargan's (1981) analysis should be a reminder that management capacity must be put in the context of political will; "a local government's capacity is its ability to do what it wants to do" (p. 652).

Much of the implementation of community-based services has been judicially mandated and accomplished in other ways over the objections of local officials acting on the types of principles outlined above. One representative of a state association of local governments pointed out that counties have little interest in implementing developmental services. However, local governments' assumption of responsibility to manage those services, even though it has not involved full fiscal responsibility, has resulted in an exponential increase in the number of employees in local human service departments. That, he noted, is a cost that is largely borne by the localities and adds to the lack of enthusiasm for community-based services on the part of many local officials. Therefore, attention to problems and perceptions of local fiscal capacity and enhancing local management capacity should not ignore the crucial dimension of local political willingness that also plays an important role.

PROBLEMS OF GOVERNANCE IN THE COMMUNITY

Conventional wisdom suggests that problems become simpler as they become more localized. Although that may be the case in some areas, it seems that managing and making decisions about human services in the community involves a degree of complexity that is not sufficiently understood (LaPorte, 1975; Parks & Ostrom, 1981). In this section of the chapter, some of the more important dimensions of this complex problem affecting developmental services at the local level are outlined, and some approaches to their resolution are described.

There are several ways in which these problems could be addressed, and no one perspective captures the full range of issues that are important because there are at least two distinct sets of dynamics at work. First, the establishment of community-based services is, in many respects, a problem of implementation. Second, the issues in the area can be approached from the perspective of problems of intergovernmental relations among federal, state, and local levels, as well as within the local government sector. In this respect, the establishment of community-based developmental services also involves a significant shift from public to private sector responsibility for delivery of services. These perspectives obviously overlap. However, if one of the most crucial concerns is indeed to identify the nature of the problem, it is important to describe how these separate frameworks each capture significant aspects of the problems of governance at the local level.

Implementing Community-Based Services

The creation of community-based services has been largely brought about through deinstitutionalization. Deinstitutionalization, whether based on court orders and decrees, plans of compliance, or other social policy foundations, is, to a large degree, a problem of implementation: "the process of carrying out authoritative public policy directives" (Nakamura & Smallwood, 1980, p. 1). The concern for the process and problems of implementation became prominent in the 1970s as the difficulties in putting the Great Society programs of the Johnson administration into practice became evident (Bardach, 1977; Nakamura & Smallwood, 1980; Pressman & Wildavsky, 1973; Rein & Rabinowitz, 1978). Many of the most important problems of implementation that these analysts identified are especially germane to the creation of community-based developmental services. Particularly relevant to this policy area is the focus on the difficulties in linkages between levels of government and types of decision-making arenas and the emphasis on the importance of communication in successful implementation. It seems that many advocates, policy-makers, and analysts fail to appreciate the extraordinary complexity of implementing at the local level those policies on the creation of community-based services that have been largely made in federal and state policy arenas.

Rein and Rabinowitz (1978) describe the problems that emerge as implementation decisions shift to different levels of government and to different decision-making frameworks. Significant problems and differences occur in the transition from the legal (judicial and legislative) domain where policy preferences are determined, to the bureaucratic area where what is administratively feasible is central, to the consensual area where the agreement of those who ultimately have a stake in the outcome is crucial (Rein & Rabinowitz, 1978). Deinstitutionalization has been characterized by these types of transitions, as state bureaucracies attempt to follow and interpret the directives of federal courts to move people from state-operated institutions to community settings and private agencies. Many of the problems that have been encountered can be seen as a result of the failure to consider the effect of different decision-making structures and processes of each level.

Nakamura and Smallwood (1980) argue that the communication linkages between the policy formulation environment and the policy implementation area are crucial elements to the success of implementation. One recent project designed to identify barriers to planning and implementation of community-based programs for children with developmental disabilities brought together a large number of local officials and key actors in the area. Approximately one-third of the 64 problems identified by this group can be characterized as involving communication between sectors and levels of government; for example, conflicting regulations, lack of awareness of the needs of clients, lack of guidelines, and lack of understanding of services by parents (Albert Einstein College of Medicine, 1986). Virtually every study of implementation has pointed to the crucial role that is played by the implementers: those public officials and key private actors who ultimately make policy at the point of delivery. The communication problem evident in the example noted here indicates that one of the significant barriers to establishing community-based developmental services is a lack of understanding of the needs, awareness of the problems involved, appreciation of the policy guidelines, and perhaps most important, consensus about the solutions on the part of key people at the point of delivery.

Intergovernmental Relations and Community Services

The complexities of intergovernmental relations are the basis of many of the problems of establishing, managing, and expanding developmental services in the community. A brief examination from this perspective indicates how some of the problems at the local level have emerged and how they might be addressed.

As in the case of a number of other problems in this area, the relative newness of the complex relationships between governments itself creates difficulties (Gargan, 1981). There has not been sufficient time to develop the "routines of politics," those well-defined procedures that simplify decisions and provide stability in the political system (Sharkansky, 1970). Many of the problems that key actors at the local level identify center on their lack of experience in this area, as well as the confusion that is often created by various federal and state policy-making bodies. For example, local officials point to the lack of coordination among planning and funding cycles between state agencies, the inconsistency in definitions of handicapping conditions and developmental disabilities, conflicting regulations, and differences in funding formulas for similar programs (Albert Einstein College of Medicine, 1986). Both the newness of the issue for local officials and the confusing array of guidelines, regulations, and funding cycles are examples of the vertical dimensions of intergovernmental relations that create difficulties at the community level.

The horizontal dimensions of the problems of intergovernmental relations present another set of concerns for local government officials and people seeking access to developmental services. In most conventional analyses of governance at the local level, there is an assumption of a unitary model of local government (Parks & Ostrom, 1981). The "government" is assumed to be a single, omniscient, and comprehensive structure for making decisions. Although the unitary assumption is not accurate at the state level, responsibility for developmental services is usually encompassed within a relatively few agencies, and decision-making extends to a similarly small number of legislative committees, executive chamber officials, and related bodies. In contrast to that comparatively simple model of state-level government, in most communities of any size responsibility for planning, budgeting, fiscal management, program operation, and quality assurance are spread among a large number of different types of local governments and quasigovernmental bodies. Few if any of those entities share the same geographic boundaries, type of client, and decision-making structure. Moreover, in contrast to different state agencies that are encompassed within one administration, many local governments and school districts function autonomously and are only loosely coupled through a variety of often tenuous linkages (LaPorte, 1975; Wieck, 1976).

This metropolitan problem has been one of the primary concerns of students of state and local governments. From the perspective of the person with a developmental disability or of his or her family, the array of services, jurisdictions, and decision-making structures and processes makes the questions of where does one go for services and who decides one is eligible extraordinarily complex. For a family with a school-age child with a developmental disability, the simple matrix illustrated in Table 6.1 of the public and services

Table 6.1. Matrix of services and providers

Service	Provider	Jurisdiction	Decision-making structure
Education	School	School district	School board
Medical services	Hospital	Health area	Board of directors
Transportation	Bus company	Metropolitan area	Transportation authority
Recreation	Town, city	Municipality	Town board, city council
Family supports	Developmental services off. (NYS)	Multi-county region	State agency
Case management	Social service department	County	County legislature, manager
Housing and day services	Private agency	Indeterminate	Board of directors

that might be required indicates the complexity of the metropolitan problem. From the perspective of local officials or state officials at the local or regional level, the metropolitan problem is a large barrier to coordination of existing services and development of new services.

It is also very important to keep in mind that deinstitutionalization and the creation of community-based services have involved a major shift from state-operated to privately operated services. The matrix of services, providers, jurisdictions, and decision-making structures takes on a qualitatively different aspect as privately provided services are added to it. Although many private agencies operate almost exclusively within the public domain through government contracts, their private character presents different types of problems in coordination, planning for new services, and quality assurance at the local level.

In New York State in the late 1970s, for example, county mental health departments, which provided developmental services, were largely concerned with mental health services. The Willowbrook Consent Decree and the ICF/MR Plan of Compliance required rapid and large-scale creation of services in the community to accomplish deinstitutionalization. The newly created Office of Mental Retardation and Developmental Disabilities bypassed county governments in many parts of the state and established these programs through direct contracts with private voluntary organizations. Doing so often involved unique contracts, reimbursement rates, and operational arrangements that provided generous incentives for those agencies, which had largely been involved in advocacy, to engage in substantial service delivery (Rothman & Rothman, 1984). Although most of these programs have since become more integrated with other local human services and are now funded through local government auspices, one state association official indicated that the vestiges of resentment left by that aggressive and singular mode of development remained a barrier to coordination at the local level.

BUILDING DEVELOPMENTAL SERVICE SYSTEMS

If the concept of a system involves, at the minimum, some interconnectedness among the various components and movement toward some common objectives, then it should be apparent that there are many substantial barriers to meeting these criteria at the local level. Local governments bear some of the costs of community-based services, particularly in increased administrative staff; provision of support services, such as recreation and transportation; and for a portion of the costs of education of handicapped children. The fiscal burden this creates for various local governments is not inconsequential. Nevertheless, it seems that coordination among the disparate elements of developmental services and integration of planning and implementation of new services are becoming more important responsibilities of local government. The major objectives of this section are to show how some of the prevailing perspectives in the field may not be facilitating coordination and integration and to examine some approaches and mechanisms that may lead to the building of local developmental service systems. The political and economic factors affecting coordination and integration are also examined because as Benson (1975) argued, "The interorganizational network may be conceived as a political economy concerned with the distribution of two scarce resources, money and authority" (p. 229).

Prevailing Views of Coordination
and Integration of Developmental Services

Coordination and integration of services have been important topics in human services delivery for some time (Gans & Horton, 1975; Morrissey, Hall, & Lindsey, 1982; National Institute of Mental Health, 1985). Cooperative efforts to arrange appropriate services for clients are regarded as crucial to the well-being of these individuals, and they are important to the organization of developmental services in the community (Elder & Magrab, 1980). However, there has been less attention paid to these efforts in the developmental services field than in such policy areas as mental health (NIMH, 1985). In some respects this is because deinstitutionalization, largely under the aegis of court orders and consent decrees, has been a more controlled process in the developmental disabilities field and has resulted in more structured residential and day program placements than has the so-called dumping of mentally ill clients from state hospitals that has contributed to the problems of the homeless that now occupy human service agencies. In any case, the thrust of much of the literature on coordination and integration, as well as some of the approaches to the problems in the developmental services field, requires that an examination of their impact on building local developmental service systems be undertaken.

Two important themes recur in the literature on coordination and integration. The first theme is the focus on gaining access to the services required to prevent institutionalization. As was pointed out in the discussion of family support services, studies of deinstitutionalized persons showed that the services required for normal community living were often unavailable or inaccessible, and their absence was related to reinstitutionalization (Bachrach, 1981; Gollay et al., 1978; Intagliata et al., 1980; Scheerenberger, 1975). These findings initially led to the creation of placement support services, and later family support service programs were developed to prevent the institutionalization of people living at home with their families. Thus, institutions constitute an important focal point in considering the need for and use of services in the community. For example, many community residential facilities for people who have been deinstitutionalized rely on the institution rather than community services for such services as transportation. From the perspective of the providers and funders of community-based services, using the institution as a provider of last resort or a source of continuing support services might prejudice their willingness to integrate the needs of deinstitutionalized persons in planning human services and to provide a full complement of services from community resources. Whatever the specific impact, it is clear that coordination and integration of community-based services cannot be considered without reference to the impact of institutions on them.

The second major theme, which is closely related to the first, is the consideration of the extent to which those services should be provided by specialized developmental service agencies or by so-called generic agencies. Both the reluctance of traditional voluntary social service agencies to serve deinstitutionalized persons with developmental disabilities (Rothman & Rothman, 1984) and the deliberate bypassing of local government mental health agencies (Castellani, Tausig, & Bird, 1984) were important factors in establishing specialized developmental service agencies at the outset of the deinstitutionalization process. In many respects, these factors contribute to the perception of dyadic relationships between specialized and generic providers. For example, Savage, Novak, and Heal (1980) argue, "Community residential facilities (CRFs) must rely on a network of community services that is prepared to adapt to the full range of human handicapping conditions" (p. 75). This view not only embodies an "us and them" perception of the organization of these services but it also is focused on deinstitutionalized persons usually in congregate care settings. Furthermore, it rests on an implicit assumption that access to generic services is often negotiated between the specialized and generic *agencies*. That view does not adequately account for the problems that the many developmentally disabled *individuals* who have never been institutionalized and are not enrolled in routine developmental services have in first gaining access to either generic or specialized developmental services.

A variation on the generic versus specialized theme is that generic services offer an improved opportunity for people with developmental disabilities. Savage, Novak, and Heal also argue, "The *vast array* of generic services, although constituting a treatment and service resource of *huge proportion*, has yet to fully meet the needs of our developmentally disabled population" (emphasis added) (1980, p. 88).

Gettings (1981) questions the utility of the generic versus specialized view of community-based services. He points out that "there are very few truly generic human service agencies," and "even those community agencies which are widely perceived to be serving the general public in actuality offer a circumscribed range of services aimed at a particular sub-group of the general population" (Gettings, 1981, p. 4). He also notes that a substantial portion of the support provided to people with developmental disabilities does indeed come from generic income maintenance, medical assistance, housing, and other sources but that people with developmental disabilities may be more successful in gaining public support under the specific disability umbrella than through general adult sources (1981).

What seems evident is that the prevailing perspective on this aspect of the coordination and integration of community services is rather limited. First, the emphasis on institutionalization seems to put a peculiar perspective on the rationale for these services and may inhibit their availability. Local governments and community agencies may continue to look to state-run institutions for supports that they would otherwise provide to dependent people in their communities. Second, the generic versus specialized perspective tends to ignore the problems of coordination among developmental service providers, often assumes an agency-to-agency linkage that ignores the problems of individuals seeking access to services, and also assumes that other services are indeed generic and plentiful when there are strong indications that they may be as "specialized" as developmental services and not as plentiful.

In general, the literature does not seem to take into account the fact that people with developmental disabilities are a rather differentiated and complex group of people who present several distinct problems of coordination and integration. It must be recognized that coordination and integration are complex issues that involve many more elements than gaining access to generic services to prevent (re)institutionalization.

The Importance of Being a Client:
Age, Income, and Institutionalization

People with developmental disabilities possess a wide range of attributes and needs that raise different problems for coordination and integration of services. The impact of these attributes on access to services is more fully discussed in Chapter 4, but a brief review here indicates their importance to the problems of coordination and integration. For example, the family with a newborn child with a developmental disability faces one set of problems of gaining access to services and arranging coordination among service providers. That same family's situation changes substantially when the child reaches school age and becomes eligible for special education and related services. Of course, their situation again changes radically when the child ages out of the education system, and the family must seek access to and attempt to coordinate a variety of adult habilitative, vocational, income mantenance, and other services. Obviously, the disabled person's age is a crucial factor in his or her eligibility for services and changes across particularly important thresholds: age 3 and age 22 significantly affect access, coordination, and integration.

Income is another demographic characteristic that is especially important in access to services. A family's low income may make it eligible for Medicaid, which may provide access to and payment for some services for a disabled family member. Low income is also a key eligibility criterion for a variety of other social welfare services, such as food stamps, housing assistance, and transportation. As an adult, a disabled person's inability to earn at a certain level may make her or him eligible for SSI.

Finally, a person's service history is a crucial situational characteristic that significantly affects access to community-based developmental services. The majority of people who have been deinstitutionalized have been placed in congregate care settings in the community, and typically, that person's day program is coordinated with his or her residential placement. Support services are often also provided to prevent reinstitutionalization (Castellani el al., 1986).

The demographic and situational characteristics discussed above are particularly important because they match eligibility criteria that provide virtually automatic or at least greatly enhanced access to services. That access often involves much more than a single transaction or tangential relationship. It typically involves becoming a client of a service provider: either a private or public agency. Often being a client of an agency for one type of service results in automatic eligibility for other services of that agency, such as family support services (Castellani et al., 1986). It may also confer virtually automatic eligibility for services or assistance from other agencies or providers, such as Medicaid eligibility for persons receiving SSI or SSDI. Most importantly from the standpoint of coordination and integration of services, being a client usually provides *organizational advocacy* for that individual; that is, the disabled individual's access to other services and their coordination and integration are very often negotiated between and among private and public agencies as transactions for their clients. It should be evident that coordination and integration of a variety of housing, vocational/habilitative, income maintenance, support, and other services are significantly enhanced when they are arranged by agency staff, rather than being left to the resources of an individual or family. Moreover, in addition to the knowledge, experience, and personal and professional relationships among agency staff, very often interagency linkages are based on statutory, fiscal, contractual, and other bases that greatly facilitate the coordination and integration of services on behalf of a client.

The fact that there are many more people with developmental disabilities living in the community than are now receiving routine and regular service as clients of service agencies indicates that there are at least two dimensions of the problem of coordination and integration of services. On the one hand, there are interorganizational relationships among agencies on behalf of their clients. On the other hand, there are a large number of disabled people and their families attempting on their own or with the assistance of such resources as protection and advocacy services to seek access. Because most community-based developmental services are routine residential and vocational/habilitative services, once an individual gains access, he or she usually becomes a long-term client. However, as more family support services become available in communities and as the intermittent and crisis needs of many developmentally disabled persons who do not participate in those routine services are addressed, the problems of one-time or intermittent access, coordination, and integration will become more apparent. Advocates and service system managers need to become much more sensitive to the fact that coordination and integration of services involves two very distinct dimensions: interorganizational relationships and individual/family attempts to gain access to and coordinate the several types of services required to live successfully in the community. Although these observations should not be surprising to most human service professionals, the approaches and mechanisms that have been employed for coordination and integration of services often do not seem to take into account the different circumstances of disabled individuals or the typical modes of current interorganizational and individual agency relationships.

Several Dimensions of Coordination and Integration

In many instances coordination of the services required in a community setting may be relatively simple because some agencies may provide a full range of residential, day habilitative, vocational, and other support and ancillary services. Gaining access to services in a comprehensive service agency may solve the problem of coordination and integration for many people with developmental disabilities. For many other people, however, day, residential, and support services may be provided by different agencies under different auspices and with different levels of complexity. Obviously, the problems of coordination and integration become increasingly complex as the number of agencies that provide services grows. Therefore, one set of problems may concern arranging the array of services that a person with developmental disabilities may need by gaining access to one comprehensive agency or through a variety of agencies.

That issue of the number of agencies involved is complicated by the fact that the providers may be federal, state, or local (including school district) governmental agencies or a variety of private voluntary and proprietary organizations. Moreover, a number of distinct types of relationships may be involved in the coordination and integration of those services. For example, application for SSI or SSDI may involve a lengthy, complex, and problematic process in order to establish eligibility. Eligibility for special education services, although not problem-free, is largely a matter of reaching school age. In other instances, state and local government agencies contract with private organizations to provide services. Access to medical and dental services in the community may involve locating a willing practitioner and convincing him or her to provide services to a person with a developmental disability. From these few examples, it should be evident that a wide range of relationships, including persuasion, contract, and statutory mandate, are involved in coordination and integration. As suggested earlier, much of the literature fails to take these important differences into account, and many of the approaches and mechanisms for coordination and integration are similarly hampered.

Providing ongoing coordination of services for a disabled person involves different concerns from managing the transition between major service domains. It is clear that the initial access to services for a person moving from special education to an adult vocational program or placement in a community residence can be a difficult and complex process involving major changes in a person's life. Arranging medical or other support services for a person who is already in a community residence and a day program obviously involves a different level of coordination and integration. Many professionals seem to fail to recognize the substantial difference between these two sets of problems.

Coordination or Capacity

As was pointed out earlier, some analysts assume that there are a "vast array" of generic services in communities (Savage et al., 1980). According to that view, the availability of community services should be enhanced by developing mechanisms of coordination and integration that will link those already existing services to people who need them. Others have argued that family support services, which were expected to be available in the community, were not present and their availability needs to be directly addressed by funders of developmental services (Castellani et al., 1986; Gollay et al., 1978).

It is unlikely that anyone will argue that the issue is solely a question of *either* increasing coordination *or* enhancing capacity. Both these approaches must be pursued to some extent in virtually any community context. Nonetheless, it is important to appreciate that assumptions about what is required to enhance the availability and accessibility of community services can have significant effects on the allocation of resources. For example, the Willowbrook Consent Decree included stipulations for substantial case management services for Willowbrook class clients placed in community settings, despite the fact that the residential, day, and ancillary services for those individuals were largely managed through other vehicles, and their community programs were highly structured, long-term arrangements (New York State Office of Mental Retardation and Developmental Disabilities, 1982). Case managers, who were assigned on a 1 : 20 ratio, therefore did not spend the majority of their time performing the ongoing service coordination and integration functions typically ascribed to case managers (Beatrice, 1980; NYS OMRDD, 1982). Because all services are costly and case management is especially expensive, this example suggests that resources that were allocated to coordination that was largely unneeded might have been used to enhance the capacity of other services.

Mechanisms for Coordination and Integration of Services

A number of mechanisms are already in place or are proposed as ways to improve the coordination and integration of developmental services. Here, three prominent approaches are examined with respect to their impact on the organization of services in the community: information and referral, case management, and single point of access.

Information and Referral (I&R)   This service is almost universally acknowledged as a mechanism for coordination and integration of services. However, this broad recognition seems to mask a failure to understand the problems, opportunities, and complexities involved with I&R. As Gargan and Shanahan (1984) have pointed out, "According to evaluations undertaken during the 1970s, I&R arrangements designed to overcome social service complexity and fragmentation had themselves become so complex and fragmented as to be counterproductive" (p. 141).

In a recent study of community support services, I&R was the most frequently offered service by the 135 provider agencies surveyed (Downey, Castellani, & Tausig, 1985). However, most of the information delivered was actually about the provider agency's own programs. Little information about other agencies was available, and there was virtually no referral to other agencies. This suggests that the agencies that are providing community-based services do not operate as a system or network of services linked by such mechanisms as information and referral.

Case Management   This is another generally acknowledged mechanism for coordination and integration of services, but is perhaps the most problematic. Virtually every discussion of case management begins with an assertion about the problems of access in a complex society. As Intagliata (1982) puts it:

> Because public funding for these programs was provided primarily through narrow categorical channels, the network of services that has resulted is highly complex, fragmented, duplicative, and uncoordinated. The barriers are particularly burdensome for those persons whose complex problems require them to engage in multiple, disconnected programs in order to get the assistance they need. (p.655)

Although there are a number of models of case management (Beatrice, 1981; Humm-Delgado, 1980), the following definition captures the essential components of this mechanism:

> Case management is a process of linking, coordinating, and monitoring various segments of a service delivery system to ensure the most comprehensive program for meeting an individual's need. (NYS OMRDD, 1982, p. 1)

Case management's role in the developmental service system poses some substantial concerns. First, many people with developmental disabilities are in highly structured congregate care residential and day programs and do not themselves face the complex and fragmented array of services that require case management. Their situations are relatively stable, and as was pointed out above, they rely on a variety of other interorganizational linkages for the coordination of their services, although case managers may be the specific individuals who handle those transactions. One study of case management activities, however, found that case managers spent relatively little of their time (about 12 percent) performing the core case management functions of linking and coordinating services (MacEachron, 1983). Most of their activities were also focused on individuals already in more structured residential and day programs. Although there are much larger numbers of people with developmental disabilities who live with their families or in independent situations, relatively few case management services were available to those individuals (MacEachron, 1983; MacEachron, Pensky, & Hawes, 1986; Commission on Quality of Care, 1984b).

Beatrice's (1981) analysis of case management is particularly relevant to this chapter because it describes the political and economic ramifications of this approach to coordination and integration. He points out that, if case management functions as it is intended, it provides the support to shift or direct lighter-care clients out of or away from institutional to noninstitutional settings. That, of course, has a problematic impact on institutional providers, including those operating more structured residential and day programs, because it lessens the cross-subsidization provided by lighter-care clients. Moreover, although many discussions of case management view such issues as referrals of clients to service providers as largely a question of communication and matching need to service, Beatrice points out that this process has important economic effects on providers who depend on those referrals of clients to stay in business and who have an economic interest in the cost of care of those clients. Successful case management requires that case managers and case management agencies have sufficient authority to make those decisions and to have them stand. The economic implications of case management are usually translated into what Beatrice terms a "political struggle" as providers attempt to use political resources to maximize gains and minimize costs associated with different types of clients (1981, p. 147).

Thus, case management, although widely acknowledged as a mechanism for coordination and integration of services, has problems that are not as widely considered. First, in the organization of community-based services, there appears to be, in some instances, an overlap of case management services for individuals who are not in situations that typically require that service. Second, case management entails important economic and political ramifications that are not usually acknowledged in discussions of its various functions and techniques. Yet, an appreciation of these dimensions is crucial to how case management is to be employed as a mechanism for coordination and integration.

Single Point of Access   The concept of a single point of access into the entire array of community-based developmental services has emerged as a possible mechanism for coordination and integration of services (Albert Einstein College of Medicine, 1986; Callahan, 1981; Diamond & Berman, 1981). In this approach, all providers and funders in an area allow one agency, interagency, or consortium-type mechanism to provide central intake, needs assessment, and assignment of clients to providers. It is obviously a powerful tool for coordination and integration of services and would address many of the concerns about inappropriate placement of clients, overlap of services, and other similar problems in local areas. Of course, the operational and perhaps fiscal efficiency that this mechanism offers is gained at the price of autonomy of the organizations that would be required to give up a substantial degree of their power to operate independently. There are some indications that agencies in some locales are willing to cede some of those functions to central bodies (Albert Einstein College of Medicine, 1986). Whether this is done to control the effects of anticipated fiscal constraints or as a result of a carefully negotiated effort to share the costs and gain the operational benefits of some centralized functions, it is clear that powerful incentives are required for agencies to give up their autonomy.

Summary

This consideration of coordination and integration of community-based services raises more questions about the organization of these services than it answers. Nonetheless, it is important because it seems that much of the literature and approaches that have been taken bring into sharper relief some important anomalies and problems that must be addressed if developmental services are to be more available and accessible.

The discussion of specialized and generic services should force the consideration of what are developmental services. Many of the services that have been provided by specialized developmental service agencies may not indeed be specific to the needs of people with developmental disabilities. Moreover, what have been often referred to as generic services may not be as plentiful or as generally available as some analysts have assumed. Longer experience in operating community-based programs and changes in the funding of the broad range of health and human services, such as block grant approaches, may bring about realignments of services and providers.

Both the generic versus specialized discussion, and studies of some of the mechanisms of coordination and integration, also show that community-based services are often oriented toward institutions and institutionalization. The organization of community-based developmental services is focused around two groups of individuals: 1) those who have been deinstitutionalized or placed from the community into congregate care residential and structured day programs and 2) those people who live on their own or with their families and need intermittent support from developmental service providers. They are not at different points on a so-called continuum of needs and services. They are two distinct groups, and their needs for service coordination are met very differently. The ways in which the coordination and integration of these services are approached clearly show the overwhelming imbalance toward those in highly structured circumstances, although the mechanisms employed are ostensibly designed for those individuals who are in more independent situations. This approach is not only costly but it works against the accessibility of services.

The discussion of some of the most prominent mechanisms employed for coordination and integration should also make it apparent that it is necessary to look beyond the questions of technique that predominate in this area. In the first instance, studies of information and referral cast serious doubt on the notion that community-based developmental services constitute a system of services or function as a part of some coherent or cohesive network.

What should also be apparent, particularly from the discussion of case management and single point of access approaches, is that mechanisms for coordination and integration are not benign in their impact on the distribution of power and money within the developmental services arena. That characterization may seem rather blunt, and it is not intended to imply that the well-being of people with developmental disabilities is not the primary consideration of advocates, providers, and policy-makers. However, a focus on coordination and integration mechanisms solely as techniques of service system management without an appreciation of their implications for the allocation of power and money in a local developmental services network is counterproductive. Organizations, no matter how laudable their objectives, tend to maintain their autonomy, seek control over their environments, and preserve and enhance their economic well-being. Mechanisms and approaches to coordinate and integrate services for people with developmental disabilities should be examined more carefully for the extent to which they affect the autonomy of service providers to select their clients, deliver their services, and maintain and maximize their political and economic position in the environment of service providers.

CONCLUSION

The most important conclusions that can be drawn from this description of problems at the point of delivery is that the community context of developmental services is extremely complex and involves several dimensions that have not been adequately addressed by advocates; federal, state, and local policy-makers; and others with a stake in the arena. That complexity has been masked to some extent because the process of deinstitutionalization has, at least at the outset, largely entailed moving people from large state-operated institutions to smaller, disaggregated facilities closer to or in population centers. That has required an enormous effort in which communities, local officials, and new types of provider organizations have participated. However, it is only recently that the extent of the problems of decision-making at the local level and the degree of complexity involved in establishing community-based developmental services that are well-managed, supported, and coordinated with other human services and resources have emerged.

It is very important to recognize that the problems of government at the local level are qualitatively different from the problems at the federal and state levels. Although federal and state policy-making involves a number of separate and often uncoordinated entities, governance at the local level encompasses an exponentially greater number of different types of governments with different jurisdictions and with distinct decision-making structures and processes. Moreover, it is at the local level that the particularly difficult problems of public and private sector relations occur. Whether an implementation, intergovernmental relations, or interorganizational perspective is employed—or more likely elements of each are combined—it is necessary that these problems and issues be addressed by an analytic framework that is more comprehensive than the relatively limited notions of preventing (re)institutionalization, gaining access to generic services, or overcoming community opposition that now seem to prevail.

Another conclusion that can be reached from this description of problems and issues at the local level is that it is crucial to examine them from the local perspective. Preventing institutionalization, gaining access to generic services, and overcoming community opposition are not local problems. Rather, fiscal responsibility for starting up, operating, and managing developmental services is the most prominently discussed problem. There are indeed some important concerns about local capacity and willingness to assume responsibility for adult services, especially in light of the federal government's failure to meet its original commitment to special education under PL 94-142. Nonetheless, there is evidence to suggest that local fiscal responsibility is not onerous and will not be an overriding barrier to further development of community-based services. What is becoming more apparent as a major problem at the local level is the lack of understanding, awareness, and knowledge about people with developmental disabilities and the services they require. In addition to the newness of the experience, the conflicting planning and funding cycles, guidelines, and regulations and ambiguous (and often absent) information about developmental services are emerging as much more important local problems (and barriers to service development) than the more salient issue of fiscal vulnerability.

These problems are closely related to another set of important local problems: the lack of managerial capacity. In contrast to the federal and state governments, local governments have not had the opportunity to develop the policy, resource, and program management capacities that must be in place if developmental services are to become community based, rather than merely located in communities.

That lack of experience in turn relates to and is indeed dependent on the resolution of the most important local level issue, the extent to which local governments and other key actors in that arena make enhancing the availability of developmental services an item on their political agenda. Developmental services must be viewed by key actors as something that they find politically expedient to pursue and an area of human services that provides them and the community more positive than negative political outcomes.

The need to rethink the approaches to coordination among various developmental services and integration with other human services is another conclusion of this chapter. Some of the ways that these issues have been addressed not only ignore several important aspects of the problem but also can lead to counterproductive efforts in this area. I&R is so generally available and assumed to be effective for coordination and integration that the failure of most efforts in this area are ignored. Case management is also widely acknowledged as an approach to coordination and integration. However, its misapplication to clients who may not require it, its cost (particularly with respect to trade-offs for greater availability), and its political consequences are also not generally recognized. Single point of access approaches are promoted for their efficiency, but the political and economic consequences have not been played out to any extent. An identification and description of the problems of coordination and integration are important if counterproductive efforts are to be avoided.

Parallel and separate developmental services are no longer fiscally or operationally tenable, nor do they contribute to integration of people with developmental disabilities into communities. Thus, it is crucial that various mechanisms and approaches be explored and tested, despite the political and economic problems in the area. Although no one mechanism emerges as a panacea, a cautious and incremental approach seems required if the complex problems are to be overcome.

Former speaker of the House of Representatives "Tip" O'Neill is reported to have said that "all politics are local." If developmental services are to become community-based, then it is imperative that analysts, advocates, and policy-makers at all levels and in all sectors become aware that the community is a qualitatively different policy context, the rules of the game are significantly distinct, and the problems to be overcome are substantially more complex than has been recognized.

7

Challenges for The Future of Community-Based Services

IN THIS CHAPTER SOME OF THE MOST SALIENT ISSUES AND THEMES OF THE book are summarized, and their implications for the future of community-based developmental services are considered. Because the field of developmental disabilities is still undergoing major changes in looking to the future, Paul Starr's (1978) caution should be heeded:

> Images of the future are usually caricatures of the present. They inflate some recognizable features of contemporary life to extravagant proportions, and out of fear or hope respond to every vagary of historical experience, as if it were a sign of destiny. (p. 81)

CONTINUING IMPACT OF HISTORY: FROM REVOLUTION TO EVOLUTION

There is simply no other area of human services in which fundamental changes in the context and structure of services, finance, clientele, and organization have been so dramatic and far-reaching in such a short period of time as in developmental disabilities. Most importantly, those changes have been almost universally positive for people with developmental disabilities, in contrast to some of the outcomes of change in other human service areas. This history, however, carries with it some problems for the future of services in this area that need to be considered.

First, the changes are not complete. There are still tens of thousands of people with developmental disabilities either living in large institutions, being inappropriately served in the community or excluded from a free and appropriate education, or receiving no services at all. In many states, virtually none of the changes described in this book have taken place. As a result, substantial amounts of the political and other kinds of energy in the field must remain devoted to the improvement of these conditions. That does not necessarily imply, however, that there is a finite store of political energy available or that attention is not being devoted to the issues raised here. Yet, in the deinstitutionalization revolution the targets are rather well-defined, the political processes familiar, and the measures of success relatively clear and demonstrable. In contrast, in the community context of services, the shape of the problems is barely emerging. The political processes are different and in some ways more complex. An entirely new set of environmental, sociodemographic, organizational, and economic factors comes into play, and the goals and objectives sought for people with developmental disabilities are more ambiguous. Moreover, it is apparent that the changes that will take place in the community will be evolutionary, rather than revolutionary. The danger is that the myriad of complex and less well-defined problems that arise in the community may not be as easily recognized or as attractive a focus of attention as the deinstitutionalization revolution.

The political ideologies that underpin advocacy and policy-making are another concern. Over the past 20 years, the paradigm has shifted from a concern for guaranteeing the procedural and substantive civil rights of people in institutions to advocacy for abolition of those institutions to ensure normalization and a least restrictive environment for people with developmental disabilities. Civil rights and normalization are simple concepts that have galvanized advocates and provided powerful guidelines for political action. Whether or not normalization is correctly interpreted in this new environment is less a concern than whether it or some other guiding principle(s) will provide the broadly acknowledged goals, clear-cut guidelines, and political energy to address the problems that people with developmental disabilities face in the community.

THE POLITICS OF ELIGIBILITY

Among the various concerns associated with who receives services, two sets of problems stand out: linking needs assessment with eligibility criteria and dealing with political boundaries of the definition of developmental disabilities, which includes maintaining a political focus for an increasingly generalized constituency.

Analysts in the field of developmental disabilities have become very sophisticated in identifying the individual, familial, situational, and environmental factors that contribute to the need for and use of services. However, it is also clear that need and use are often unrelated. For some time to come, prior institutionalization will continue to act as a "wild card" factor for access. In addition, however, there are several other factors, including age, sex, income, race, and geography, that often have idiosyncratic effects on access to services that are largely unrelated to specific needs. The extent to which anomalous and discrepant factors continue to influence access will undermine the overall credibility and political currency of advocates for more services. Moreover, this becomes more of a potential problem as services shift from public to private provision and the linkages for ensuring equity of access become more indirect and tenuous.

A more practical, but nonetheless important, aspect of the problem of linking need and eligibility is translating those needs assessments into decision criteria for managers in the community. The wide variety of factors that influence access to services is usually taken into account in decisions for out-of-home placement or entrance into other long-term services. However, many of the services that are emerging in community contexts are one-time, intermittent, short-term, or substantially different from traditional residential and day services. The need for valid, reliable, and easily applied criteria for access to these community-based developmental services will become increasingly important.

The second set of problems concerns the political boundaries of the definition of developmental disabilities. One aspect is the types of disabilities that are deemed to be "developmental." In many respects, community-based developmental services are attractive alternatives to no services or services in other arenas for people with mental and physical disabilities closely related to mental retardation. Advocates for an increasing number of disability groups have sought access to these services. However, funders of developmental services seek to limit access, as in the case of the Health Care Finance Administration's decision to reclassify autism as a mental illness and exclude people with that disability from ICFs/MR. In addition, advocates for people with more traditional developmental disabilities often view the increase in the types of disabilities encompassed in the definition with concern for the effect of more people competing for limited resources.

The political ramifications of the functional definition of developmental disabilities is the second aspect of the boundary issue. A focus on the functional components of developmental disabilities, coupled with a trend toward greater coordination among human services in the community, will lead to increasing reorganization of human services around the similar service needs of various dependent populations. This may be a positive development both from the standpoint of a fuller integration of people with developmental disabilities into communities and from the perspective of service efficiency and cost effectiveness. However, the political power of a developmental disability constituency may be diminished when submerged into a broader dependent population group, including the elderly and the chronically mentally ill, who have many of the same functional deficits. The political power of the former group (elderly citizens) is based on very large numbers, and their interests may predominate. The latter group, that is, individuals with chronic mental illness, seems to have little political power, and the political power of advocates for people with developmental disabilities may be diminished when associated with the problems and needs of that group.

In general, both traditional and new models of community-based developmental services are attractive for people with disabilities. Previously unserved people, those now in other less-desirable service settings, and people who had not been considered developmentally disabled are seeking access to them. There are serious deficiencies in the capacity to make rational, equitable, and politically defensible choices about who is served. These problems will undercut the political credibility of advocates for more services, and correcting them should be given a very high priority on both the political and professional agenda. Moreover, advocates for people with developmental disabilities face difficult political choices with respect to their inclusion with other dependent groups in the community. Local government managers are increasingly looking for more efficient and cost-effective ways of delivering human services. The political costs and benefits of generic and integrated solutions to the needs of dependent populations may not satisfy advocates for people with developmental disabilities.

ORGANIZATION OF COMMUNITY-BASED SERVICES

For many people, deinstitutionalization and the creation of community-based services have brought services closer to population centers and placed smaller residential and day programs at different sites. These services are often provided by comprehensive agencies that deliver the complete range of services and supports. These changes have usually been positive for people with developmental disabilities. However, the community environment has brought about changes in what had been total care programs and has given rise to entirely new types of services. These changes have been so significant that they require a fundamental re-examination of the organization of community-based services.

The first question raised by many of the changes that have occurred is; *What are developmental services?* The term has been used throughout the book as a convenient way of referring to the range of services and supports that people with developmental disabilities need to live successful, normal lives. It is important, however, to consider whether developmental services are a part of a coherent and integrated disciplinary, professional framework. There may be a core of clinical services that meet those criteria. However, it is obvious that major services used by people with developmental disabilities fall within educational, vocational rehabilitation, income maintenance, housing, medical, social service, and other human service domains. Moreover, in those domains, people with developmental disabilities are a small segment of the people served, so that their specific needs do not have a major impact on the definition of those fields. Therefore, developmental services may be defined more by the people served and the organizations providing the services than by the unique character of the services themselves. That may be a very important consideration when the impact of environmental factors and other policy initiatives on developmental services organizations is considered.

In many states, there have been major shifts from institutional care to community-based programs and changes in developmental service programs in those communities. The focus on vocational services and the emergence of a variety of innovative programs are substantial steps toward enabling people with developmental disabilities to lead more normal lives. Such service models as family support services are especially significant because they are unique to the community context and represent entirely new approaches to the needs of people with disabilities. These services are often in a variety of community locations—work sites, apartment houses, family homes—that are more dispersed than the congregate care settings typical of many traditional developmental service programs. They involve types of services and mechanisms—job coaches, regular wages, vouchers, home attendants—that are not only new to the developmental services field but also serve to decrease the dependence of people with disabilities and their families on traditional developmental service agencies. Moreover, these new and changed service models have brought many new people into the developmental services arena: individuals who are less disabled, family members, people with disabilities other than mental retardation, and families with 10 or so years of experience dealing with schools. In general, the dispersal of services, the closer links to other human services and supports, the new mechanisms for securing services, and the new clientele are likely to have an important impact on the agencies that provide developmental services and the overall organization of services in communities.

COMMUNITY-BASED DECISION-MAKING

Deinstitutionalization and the subsequent establishment of services in communities are major social policy phenomena, and it is naive to believe that changes of that magnitude are brought about without a great deal of opposition and consternation. Much of that has been expressed by neighbors of community-based agencies, local government officials, established social service agencies, and others in communities who have been closest to the changes. Community residences have been imposed on neighborhoods over the objections of neighbors by taking away from local officials some traditional zoning and housing prerogatives. Human service agencies in some communities have been bypassed to establish new provider organizations, and incentives for program development have upset the balance between local governments and other provider organizations. Children have been provided special education and related services despite the (correct) contention by administrators and school boards that funding for these services has not kept pace with mandates. In many ways this situation will continue. Therefore, one of the biggest challenges facing the field of developmental disabilities is to make developmental services truly community-based, rather than merely located in communities, despite the problems of the sort outlined here.

Although the local share of the costs of special education remains a problem, it does not appear that local fiscal capacity will be a major barrier to enhancing the availability of developmental services. The capacity of communities to manage developmental services seems to be a much greater challenge. The myriad of services within the developmental framework results in a complex and often incompatible array of funding formulas and cycles, policy guidelines, service definitions, and eligibility criteria that confound the efforts of local government officials and other key actors to plan for, manage, and coordinate these services. In addition to those concerns, the so-called metropolitan problem presents an enormous barrier to establishing local developmental service systems. Coordination among a variety of different local governmental bodies with overlapping jurisdictions and distinct decision-making structures, as well as with private sector organizations, requires much greater expertise and effort than has been expected and supported by federal and state officials. The experience at the local level is also causing a re-examination of some notions about coordination and integration of services. Problems with the overall approach, as well as such specific mechanisms as information and referral and case management, indicate that new approaches and mechanisms of coordination and integration need to be developed.

The most important issue in the local arena concerns political will. If developmental services are to become truly community-based, then they must do what communities want them to do. They must be on the local political agenda in much the same way as schools and highways and must be seen as services and resources that people in those communities want and local officials find politically attractive. If federal and state governments do indeed absorb most of the costs of developmental services, and if recognition and support are given to the problems of management capacity, then local government officials and other key actors can turn their attention to ways of making developmental services community-based.

POLITICAL ECONOMY OF DEVELOPMENTAL DISABILITIES

Courts, legislatures, and public bureaucracies at the federal, state, and local levels have been the focus of demands by advocates for reform, and the changes in the size and structure of community-based developmental services have been achieved through those institutions of public policy. Public policy will certainly remain the primary framework within which deinstitutionalization continues and community-based services evolve. This book has shown, however, that policy-making at the local level is a very different and, in many ways, more complex policy arena in which new actors, decision-making structures, processes, and environmental factors come into play. The amount of developmental services in communities, how they are organized and delivered, who receives them, and how their costs are allocated and benefits distributed are also the outcomes of economic as well as political processes.

Of course, the economic dimensions of developmental services are closely related, indeed linked in almost all respects, to public policy. Nonetheless, they have become sufficiently distinct and important that they merit much more attention than they have been given to this point in the evolution of community-based services.

This book has explored many of the specific topics that are central to the economics of developmental disabilities. However, more important than the specific topics is the perspective that a focus on these issues brings.

One of the most important features of that perspective is a broader awareness of the roles of individuals, families, providers, and others as economic actors. Much of the literature in the field assumes that people with developmental disabilities, their families, and the private agencies that provide services are relatively passive actors in the developmental disabilities arena. People with disabilities are clients, families are advocates, and providers are certified, inspected, and contracted. Although in the language of the political systems model, inputs are demands, the typical positions of clients, families, and providers are cast in those passive or, at best, reactive roles.

At a basic level, economics concerns exchange. Many of the types of activities and factors described in this book can be better understood and their impact assessed from that fundamental perspective of economics. When people with disabilities increasingly work for regular wages outside sheltered environments, when families are empowered to purchase services through such mechanisms as vouchers and cash subsidies, and when private agencies begin to act more as an industry than as advocates who also happen to be providers, then the perspectives of economics must be employed if the consequences of those roles and activities are to be understood.

Economics also concerns money. Advocates, analysts, and policy-makers seem to have come to grips with the use of political power. It is generally understood and appreciated that court orders, statutes, appropriations, regulations, and the other public policy outputs that serve to achieve the objectives of social policy are brought about through the exercise of political power. Advocates have become increasingly astute, aggressive, and unapologetic about exercising it. However, these same people seem less comfortable with the notion that the more than $15 billion of public expenditures and probably several times that amount in private expenditures create significant economic dynamics that are related to, but not entirely concerned with, the well-being of people with developmental disabilities. That is, people with disabilities, families, provider agencies, employees, and communities have important economic interests in the expenditure of those funds. Although their concern for the needs of people with developmental disabilities may or may not be paramount, their activities as employees, employers, taxpayers, and corporations also have a significant, independent impact on the amount of developmental services in a community and the ways in which they are organized, financed, and delivered.

The impact of those political and economic factors on the availability and accessibility of community-based services must be assessed. A perspective that either ignores the effects of these roles and activities or regards them as somehow illegitimate is limited and counterproductive. People with developmental disabilities, their families, employers, service organizations, and governments function within a complex political and economic environment. Political economy is a framework that contributes to an understanding of the central factors and processes at work and an appreciation of their important consequences for people with developmental disabilities.

References

Abad, R. J., Ramos, J., & Boyce, E. (1974). A model for delivery of mental health services to Spanish speaking minorities. *American Journal of Orthopsychiatry, 44,* 584–595.

Abeson, A., & Zettel, J. (1977). The end of the quiet revolution: The Education for All Handicapped Children Act of 1975. *Exceptional Children, 44,* 114–128.

Accountants for the Public Interest. (1983). *The transfer of people versus dollars: Intergovernmental financing for mental health services in the State of New York.* New York: Author.

Aday, L., Chin, G., & Anderson, R. (1980). Methodological issues in health care surveys of the Spanish heritage population. *American Journal of Public Health, 70,* 367–374.

Agosta, J. M., & Bradley, V. J. (1985a). Family based care and social policy: Recommendations for change. In J. M. Agosta & V. J. Bradley (Eds.), *Family care for persons with developmental disabilities: A growing commitment* (pp. 252–263). Boston: Human Services Research Institute.

Agosta, J. M., & Bradley, V. J. (Eds.). (1985b). *Family care for persons with developmental disabilities: A growing commitment.* Boston: Human Services Institute.

Agosta, J. M., & Bradley, V. J. (1985c). Using tax policy in support of families who have a member with developmental disabilities. In J. M. Agosta & V. J. Bradley (Eds.), *Family care for persons with developmental disabilities: A growing commitment* (pp. 165–183). Boston: Human Services Research Institute.

Agosta, J., Bradley, V. J., Jennings, D., Feinberg, B., & Gettings, R. (1984). *Family support programs for families with members who are developmentally disabled: Review of the literature with an emphasis on financial assistance strategies.* Boston: Human Services Research Institute.

Agosta, J. M., Bradley, V. J., Rugg, A., Spence, R., & Covert, S. (1985). *Designing programs to support family care for persons with developmental disabilities: Concepts to practice.* Boston: Human Services Research Institute.

Agosta, J. M., Jennings, D., & Bradley, V. (1985). Statewide family support programs: National survey results. In J. M. Agosta & V. J. Bradley (Eds.), *Family care for persons with developmental disabilities: A growing commitment* (pp. 94–112). Boston: Human Services Research Institute.

Aird, R. B., Masland, R. L., & Woodbury, D. M. (1984). *The epilepsies: A critical review.* New York: Raven Press.

Albert Einstein College of Medicine. (1986). *Long range planning for community-based services for disabled and at risk children (0-5) and their families in Monroe County, New York: A task force report.* Bronx, New York: Author.

Bachrach, L. L. (1981). A conceptual approach to deinstitutionalization of the mentally retarded: A perspective from the experience of the mentally ill. In R. H. Bruininks, C. Meyers, B. Sigford, & K. C. Lakin (Eds.), *Deinstitutionalization and community adjustment of mentally retarded people* (pp. 51–67). Washington, DC: American Association on Mental Deficiency.

Bachrach, L. L. (1985). Deinstitutionalization: The meaning of the least restrictive alternative. In R. H. Bruininks & K. C. Lakin (Eds.), *Living and learning in the least restrictive environment* (pp. 23–36). Baltimore: Paul H. Brookes Publishing Co.

Bahl, R. (1984). *Financing state and local government in the 1980's.* New York: Oxford University Press.

Baldwin, C. Y., & Bishop, C. (1984). Return to nursing home investment: Issues for public policy. *Health Care Financing Review 5,* 43–52.

Bangser, M. R. (1985). *Lessons in transitional employment: The demonstration for mentally retarded workers.* New York: Manpower Demonstration Research Corporation.

Bank-Mikkelson, N. E. (1969). A metropolitan area in Denmark: Copenhagen. In R. Kugel & W. Wolfensberger (Eds.), *Changing patterns in residential services for the mentally retarded.* Washington, DC: President's Committee on Mental Retardation.

Bardach, E. (1977). *The implementation game.* Cambridge, MA: M.I.T. Press.

Bates, M. V. (1983). *State family support/cash subsidy programs.* Madison, WI: Wisconsin Council on Developmental Disabilities.

Bates, M. V. (1985). *State zoning legislation: A purview.* Madison, WI: Wisconsin Council on Developmental Disabilities.

Beatrice, D. F. (1980). *Case management: A policy option for long term care.* Washington, DC: Health Care Financing Administration.

Beatrice, D. F. (1981). Case management: A policy option for long term care. In J. J. Callahan Jr. & S. S. Wallack (Eds.), *Reforming the long term care system.* Lexington, MA: Lexington Books.

Benson, J. K. (1975). The interorganizational network as a political economy. *Administrative Science Quarterly, 20,* 229–249.

Berger, M., & Foster, M. (1986). Applications of family therapy theory to research and interventions with families with mentally retarded children. In J. J. Gallagher & P. M. Vietze (Eds.), *Families of handicapped persons: Research, programs, and policy issues* (pp. 251–260). Baltimore: Paul H. Brookes Publishing Co.

Berkowitz, M., Johnson, W. G., & Murphy, E. H. (1976). *Public policy towards disability.* New York: Praeger.

Beziat, C., & Pell, K. (1985). Marketing innovative vocational programming in rehabilitation facilities. In National Association of Rehabilitation Facilities (Ed.), *From theory to implementation: A guide to supported employment for rehabilitation facilities* (pp. 47–73). Washington, DC: Author.

Bird, W. A. (1984a). *A survey of family support programs in seventeen states.* Albany: New York State Office of Mental Retardation and Developmental Disabilities.

Bird, W. A. (1984b). *Sources of funding for day programs.* Albany: New York State Office of Mental Retardation and Developmental Disabilities.

Bird, W. A. (1984c). *Prevention programs.* Albany: New York State Office of Mental Retardation and Developmental Disabilities.

Birnbaum, H., Burke R., Swearingen, C., and Dunlop, B. (1984). Implementing community-based long term care: Experience of New York's long term home health care program. *The Geronotologist 24*(4), 380–386.

Bishop, C. E. (1981). A compulsory national long term care insurance program. In J. J. Callahan Jr. & S. S. Wallack (Eds.), *Reforming the long term care system* (pp. 61–93). Lexington, MA: Lexington Books.

Blacher, J. (1984). *Severely handicapped young children and their families.* New York: Academic Press.

Black, M. M., Small, M. W., Crites, L. S., & Sachs, M. L. (1986). *Mentally retarded adults and their families: A model of stress and urgency.* Baltimore: University of Maryland School of Medicine.

Blackwell, J. E. (1975). *The black community: Diversity and unity.* New York: Dodd, Mead & Company.

Boggs, E. M. (1979). Economic factors in family care. In R. H. Bruininks & G. C. Krantz (Eds.), *Family care of developmentally disabled members: Conference proceedings* (pp. 47–60). Minneapolis, MN: University of Minnesota.

Boggs, E. M. (1981). Behavioral fisics. In J. J. Bevilacqua (Ed.), *Changing government policies for the mentally disabled* (pp. 39–100). Cambridge, MA: Ballinger Publishing Co.

Boggs, E., Lakin, K. C., & Clauser, S. (1985). Medicaid coverage of residential services. In K. C. Lakin, B. Hill, & R. H. Bruininks (Eds.), *An analysis of Medicaid's Intermediate Care Facility for the Mentally Retarded (ICF/MR Program)* (pp. 1-1–1-78). Minneapolis, MN: Center for Residential and Community Services, University of Minnesota.

Braddock, D. (1981). Deinstitutionalization of the retarded: Trends in public policy. *Hospital and Community Psychiatry, 32,* 607.

Braddock, D. (1986). From Roosevelt to Reagan: Federal spending analysis for mental retardation and developmental disabilities. *American Journal of Mental Deficiency, 90,*(5), 479–489.

Braddock, D. (1987). *Federal policy toward mental retardation and developmental disabilities.* Baltimore: Paul H. Brookes Publishing Co.

Braddock, D., & Heller, T. (1985). The closure of mental retardation facilities: Trends in the United States. *Mental Retardation, 24*(4), 168–176.

Braddock, D., & Hemp, R. (1985). *Intergovernmental spending for mental retardation in the United States* (Public Policy Monograph No. 16). Chicago: Institute for the Study of Developmental Disabilities.

Braddock, D., & Hemp, R. (1986). Governmental spending for mental retardation, 1977-1984. *Hospital and Community Psychiatry, 37*(7), 702–707.

Braddock, D., Hemp, R., & Howes, R. (1984). *Public expenditures for mental retardation and developmental disabilities in the United States* (Public Policy Monograph Series No. 5). Chicago: Institute for the Study of Developmental Disabilities.

Braddock, D., Hemp, R., & Howes, R. (1985a). *Costs of institutional care in* the United States (Public Policy Monograph No. 12). Chicago: Institute for the Study of Developmental Disabilities.

Braddock, D., Hemp, R., & Howes, R. (1985b). Financing community services in the United States: An analysis of trends (Public Policy Monograph No. 13). Chicago: Institute for the Study of Developmental Disabilities.

Braddock, D., Hemp, R., & Howes, R. (1985c). Public expenditures for mental retardation and developmental disabilities in the United States: Analytic summary (Public Policy Monograph No. 6). Chicago: Institute for the Study of Developmental Disabilities.

Braddock, D., Hemp, R., & Howes, R. (1986). Costs of institutional care in the United States. Mental Retardation, 24, 9–17.

Bradley, V. J. (1981). Mental disabilities services: Maintenance of public accountability in a privately operated system. In J. J. Bevilacqua (Ed.), Changing government policies for the mentally disabled (pp. 193–208). Cambridge, MA: Ballinger Publishing Co.

Bradley, V. J. (1985). Implementation of court and consent decrees: Some current lessons. In R. H. Bruininks & K. C. Lakin (Eds.), Living and learning in the least restrictive environment (pp. 81–96). Baltimore: Paul H. Brookes Publishing Co.

Brancato, F. (1985, November 7). Workers in New York State foster-care agencies need support [Letter to the editor]. New York Times, p. A20.

Brecher, C., & Knickman, J. (1985). A reconsideration of long term care policy. Journal of Health Politics, Policy and Law, 10(2), 245–273.

Brown, L. D., Fossett, J. W., & Palmer, K. T. (1984). The changing politics of federal grants. Washington, DC: The Brookings Institution.

Bruininks, R. H. (1979). The needs of families. In R. H. Bruininks & G. C. Krantz (Eds.), Family care of developmentally disabled members: Conference proceedings (pp. 3–10). Minneapolis, MN: University of Minnesota.

Bruininks, R. H., & Krantz, G. C. (1979). Family care of developmentally disabled members: Conference proceedings. Minneapolis, MN: University of Minneapolis.

Bruininks, R. H., & Lakin, K. C. (1985). Perspectives and prospects for social and educational integration. In R. H. Bruininks & K. C. Lakin (Eds.), Living and learning in the least restrictive environment (pp. 263–277). Baltimore: Paul H. Brookes Publishing Co.

Bruininks, R. H., Meyers, C., Edward, S., Barbara B., & Lakin, K. C. (Eds.). (1981). Deinstitutionalization and community adjustment of mentally retarded people (Monograph No. 4). Washington, DC: American Association on Mental Deficiency.

Bryce, H. J. (1985, October). New directions in the education of managers of non-profit organizations. Paper presented at the meeting of the Association for Public Policy Analysis and Management, Washington, DC.

Buehler, B. A., Menolascino, F. J., & Stark, J. A. (1986). Medical care of individuals with developmental disabilities: Future implications. In W. E. Kiernan & J. A. Stark (Eds.), Pathways to employment for adults with developmental disabilities (pp. 241–249). Baltimore: Paul H. Brookes Publishing Co.

Burtless, G. T. (1985). Are targeted wage subsidies harmful?: Evidence from a wage voucher experiment. *Industrial and Labor Relations Review, 39*(1), 105–114.

Burtless, G. T. (1986, January 7). Jobs tax credit stigmatizes disadvantaged workers [Letter to the editor]. *New York Times,* p. A30.

Business Coalition for Fair Competition. (1985). *Unfair competition in the states: How to combat competition from non-profit business ventures.* Washington, DC: Author.

Callahan, J. J., Jr. (1981). Single agency option for long term care. In J. J. Callahan, Jr. & S. S. Wallack (Eds.), *Reforming the long term care system* (pp. 163–183). Lexington, MA: Lexington Books.

Callahan, J. J., Jr., & Wallack, S. S. (1981). Major reforms in long term care. In J. J. Callahan, Jr. & S. S. Wallack (Eds.), *Reforming the long term care system* (pp. 3–9). Lexington, MA: Lexington Books.

Campbell, J. F. (1985). Supported work approaches for the traditional rehabilitation facility. In National Association of Rehabilitation Facilities (Eds.), *From theory to implementation: A guide to supported employment for rehabilitation facilities* (pp. 1–20). Washington, DC: Author.

Castellani, P. J. (1975). *The impact of judicial outputs on mental hygiene in New York State.* Unpublished doctoral dissertation, Syracuse University.

Castellani, P. J. (1985). Policy options for family support services. In V. J. Bradley & J. Agosta (Eds.), *Family care for persons with developmental disabilities* (pp. 114–148). Boston: Human Services Research Institute.

Castellani, P. J. (1986). Policy perspectives in the new environment of developmental services. *Mental Retardation, 24*(1), 5–7.

Castellani, P. J., Downey, N. A., Tausig, M. B., & Bird, W. A. (1986). Availability and accessibility of family support services. *Mental Retardation, 24*(2), 71–79.

Castellani, P. J., & Puccio, P. S. (1984). *The development of family support services for the developmentally disabled: An administrative and political perspective.* Paper presented at the American Society for Public Administration National Conference, Denver.

Castellani, P. J., Tausig, M., & Bird, W. (1984). Structural and contextual factors affecting advocacy for community support services. In J. A. Mulick & B. L. Mallory (Eds.), *Transitions in mental retardation: Advocacy, technology and science* (pp. 16–41). Norwood, NJ: Ablex Publishing Corp.

Chernish, W. A., Britt, B., Nutter, S. O., & Sakry, L. A. (1985). Components of a supported work model for private rehabilitation facilities. In National Association of Rehabilitation Facilities (Ed.), *From theory to implementation: A guide to supported employment for rehabilitation facilities* (pp. 21–45). Washington, DC: Author.

Chubb, J. E. (1985) The political economy of federalism. *American Political Science Review, 79*(4), 994–1015.

Clark, T. N. (1985). Fiscal strain: How different are snow belt cities and sun belt cities? In P. E. Peterson (Ed.), *The new urban reality* (pp. 253–280). Washington, DC: The Brookings Institution.

Clauser, S. B. (1985, October). Recent trends in Medicaid coverage of long term residential care for the mentally retarded: Implications for policy research. Paper presented at the meeting of the Association for Public Policy Analysis and Management, Washington, DC.

Cohen, H. J. (1975). Obstacles to developing community services for mentally retarded. In M. J. Begab and S. A. Richardson (Eds.), *The mentally retarded and society: A social science perspective* (pp. 401–421). Baltimore: University Park Press.

Cohen, H. J. (1979). Community health planning. In P. R. Magrab & J. O. Elder (Eds.), *Planning for services to handicapped persons: Community, education, health* (pp. 91–120). Baltimore: Paul H. Brookes Publishing Co.

Cohen, S., Semmes, M., & Guralnick, J. (1979). Public Law 94–142 and the education of pre-school handicapped children. *Exceptional Children, 45,* 279–284.

Coleman, R. (1980). Minorities and mental retardation services in the Bronx. In H. J. Cohen & D. Kligler (Eds.), *Urban community care for the developmentally disabled* (pp. 60–67). Springfield, IL: Charles C Thomas.

Comegys, A. (1985). A parent's perspective. In J. M. Agosta & V. J. Bradley (Eds.), *Family care for persons with developmental disabilities: A growing commitment* (pp. 18–33). Boston: Human Services Research Institute.

Commission on Quality of Care for the Mentally Disabled (NYS). (1984a). *Pitfalls in the community-based system.* Albany: Author.

Commission on Quality of Care for the Mentally Disabled (NYS). (1984b). *Promoting equity in the family of New York: A review of outpatient services for developmentally disabled people.* Albany: Author.

Conley, R. W. (1965). *The economics of vocational rehabilitation.* Baltimore: The Johns Hopkins University Press.

Conley, R. W. (1973). *The economics of mental retardation.* Baltimore: Johns Hopkins University Press.

Conley, R. W. (1985). Impact of federal programs on employment of mentally retarded persons. In K. C. Lakin & R. H. Bruininks (Eds.), *Strategies for achieving community integration of developmentally disabled citizens* (pp. 193–216). Baltimore: Paul H. Brookes Publishing Co.

Conley, R. W., & Noble, J. H., Jr. (1985, April). *Several handicapped Americans: Victims of misguided policies.* Paper presented at the meeting on Economics of Disability, U.S. Department of Education, Washington, DC.

Conley, R. W., Noble, J. H., Jr., & Elder, J. K. (1986). Problems with the service system. In W. E. Kiernan & J. A. Stark (Eds.), *Pathways to employment for adults with developmental disabilities* (pp. 67–83). Baltimore: Paul H. Brookes Publishing Co.

Conroy, J. W., & Bradley, V. J. (1985). *The Pennhurst longitudinal study: A report of five years of research and analysis.* Philadelphia: Temple University Developmental Disabilities Center.

Cook, J. R. (1985, October). *What are the most serious problems in non-profit organizations: A practitioner's perspective.* Paper presented at the meeting of the Association for Public Policy Analysis and Management, Washington, DC.

Covington v. Harris, 325 F. Supp. 325 (1969).

Dana, R. H. (1981). *Human services for cultural minorities.* Baltimore: University Park Press.

Dawson, R. E., & Robinson, J. A. (1963). Inter-party competition, economic variables and welfare policies in the American states. *Journal of Politics, 25,* 265–289.

DeJong, G. (1979). Independent living: From social movement to analytic paradigm. *Archives of Physical Medicine Rehabilitation, 60,* 435–446.

DeJong, G., & Wenker, T. (1979). Attendant care as a prototype independent living service. *Archives of Physical Medicine Rehabilitation, 60,* 477–482.

Derrico, E. (1982). *The evolution of mental health policy and the homeless: Policy as its own cause.* Unpublished manuscript, State University at New York, Department of Political Science, Albany.

Deutsch, A. (1949). *The mentally ill in America: A history of their care and treatment from colonial times.* New York: Columbia University Press.

Diamond, L. M., & Berman, D. E. (1981). The social/health maintenance organization: A single entry, prepaid, long term care delivery system. In J. J. Callahan and S. S. Wallack (Eds.), *Reforming the long term care system* (pp. 185–213). Lexington, MA: Lexington Books.

Dolan, L. W., & Wolpert, J. (1982). *Long term neighborhood property impacts of group homes for mentally retarded people.* Princeton, NJ: Princeton University Woodrow Wilson School of Public and International Affairs.

Downy, N. A., Castellani, P. J., & Tausig, M. B. (1985). The provision of information and referral services in the community. *Mental Retardation, 23*(1), 21–25.

Dunlap, W. R. (1976). Services for families of the developmentally disabled. *Social Work, 21,* 220–223.

Dunst, C. J. (1985). Overview of the efficacy of early intervention programs: Methodological and conceptual considerations. In L. Brickman & D. Weatherford (Eds.), *Evaluating early intervention programs for severely handicapped children and their families,* Austin, TX: PRO-ED

Dunst, C. J., & Rheingrover, R. M. (1981). Analysis of the efficacy of infant intervention programs for handicapped children. *Evaluation and Program Planning, 4,* 287–323.

Dybwad, G. (1966). *The mentally retarded child under five.* Arlington, VA: Association for Retarded Citizens.

Dye, T. R. (1966). *Politics, economics and the public: Policy outcomes in the American states.* Chicago, Rand-McNally.

Easton, D. (1957). An approach to the analysis of political systems. *World Politics, 9,* 383–400.

Easton, D. (1965). *A framework for political analysis.* Englewood Cliffs, NJ: Prentice-Hall.

Edgar, E., & Heinowski, J. (1985). In partnership with families: The role of rehabilitation professionals in working with families of persons with disabilities. In National Association of Rehabilitation Facilities (Ed.), *From theory to implementation: A guide to supported employment for rehabilitation facilities* (pp. 85–93). Washington, DC: Author.

Edmundson, K. (1985). The discovery of siblings. *Mental Retardation 23*(2), 49–51.

Elder, J. O. (1979). Coordination of service delivery systems. In P. R. Magrab & J. O. Elder (Eds.) *Planning for services to handicapped persons: Community, education, health* (pp. 193–209). Baltimore, Paul H. Brookes Publishing Co.

Elder, J. O., & Magrab, P. R. (Eds.). (1980). *Coordinating services to handicapped children: A handbook for interagency collaboration.* Baltimore: Paul H. Brookes Publishing Co.

Ellien, V. (1985). The benchwork model of supported employment. In National Association of Rehabilitation Facilities (Ed.), *From theory to imple-*

mentation: A guide to supported employment for rehabilitation facilities (pp. 75–84). Washington, DC: Author.

Eyman, R. K., Boroskin, A., & Hostetter, S. (1977). Use of alternative living plans for developmentally disabled children by minority parents. Mental Retardation, 15, 21–23.

Farber, B. (1968). Mental retardation: Its social context and social consequences. Boston: Houghton Mifflin.

Fernald, C. D. (1984). Too little too late: Deinstitutionalization and the development of community services for mentally retarded people. Chapel Hill, NC: Bush Institute for Child and Family Policy, University of North Carolina.

Fernald, C. D. (1986). Changing Medicaid and intermediate care facilities for the mentally retarded (ICF/MR): Evaluation of alternatives. Mental Retardation, 24(1), 36–42.

Frankfather, D. L., Smith, M. J., & Caro, F. G. (1983). Designs for home care entitlements. In R. Perlman (Ed.), Family home care: Critical issues for services and policies (pp. 264–279). New York: The Haworth Press.

Friedman, J. R., & Daly, R. W. (1973, Spring). Civil commitment and the doctrine to balance: A critical analysis. Santa Clara Lawyer, 13.

Gallagher, J. J., Beckman, P., & Cross, A. H. (1983). Families of handicapped children: Sources of stress and its amelioration. Exceptional Children, 50(1), 10–19.

Gallagher, J. J., & Vietze, P. M. (Eds.). (1986). Families of handicapped persons: Research, programs, and policy issues. Baltimore: Paul H. Brookes Publishing Co.

Galvin, D. E. (1982). Rehabilitation of the severely handicapped, PL 93-112: A retrospective appraisal by a state vocational rehabilitation director. In J. Rubin (Ed.), Alternatives in rehabilitating the handicapped: A policy analysis. New York: Human Sciences Press.

Gans, S., & Horton, G. (1975). Integration of human services: The state and municipal levels. New York: Praeger.

Gardner, J. F. (1986). Implementation of the home and community-based waiver. Mental Retardation, 24(1), 18–26.

Gargan, J. J. (1981, November/December). Consideration of local government capacity. Public Administration Review, 649–658.

Gargan, J. J. (1985). Fiscal dependency and governmental capacity in American cities. In J. Rabin & D. Dodd (Eds.), State and local government administration (pp. 187–212). New York: Marcel Dekker Inc.

Gargan, J. J., & Moore, C. M. (1984, November/December). Enhancing local government capacity in budget decision making: The use of group process techniques. Public Administration Review, pp. 504–511.

Gargan, J. J., & Shanahan, J. L. (1984). Model I & R systems in the United States: Public policy issues in capacity building. In R. W. Levinson & K. S. Hayes (Eds.), Accessing human services: International perspectives (pp. 141–170). Beverly Hills, CA: Sage Publications.

Gettings, R. M. (1980, October 24). Federal financing of services to mentally retarded persons: Current issues and policy options. Alexandria, VA: National Association of State Mental Retardation Program Directors.

Gettings, R. M. (1981). Generic vs. specialized services: The ying and yang of programming for developmentally disabled clients. Alexandria, VA: National Association of State Mental Retardation Program Directors.

Gilbert, N. (1983). *Capitalism and the welfare state: Dilemmas of social benevolence.* New Haven, CT: Yale University Press.

Gliedman, J., & Roth, W. (1980). *The unexpected minority: Handicapped children in America.* New York: Harcourt Brace Jovanovich.

Gold, S. D. (1983). *State and local fiscal relations in the early 1980's.* Washington, DC: The Urban Institute Press.

Gollay, E., Freedman, R., Wyngaarden, M., & Kurtz, N. R. (1978). *Coming back.* Cambridge, MA: Abt Books.

Grossman, H. J. (1983). *Classification in mental retardation.* Washington, DC: American Association on Mental Deficiency.

Halderman & Pennhurst State School and Hospital, 446 F. Supp. 1295 (1978).

Hansmann, H. B. (1980). The role of nonprofit enterprise. *Yale Law Journal, 89*(5), 835–901.

Hansmann, H. (1981). Why are nonprofit organizations exempted from corporate income taxation? In M. I. White (Ed.), *Nonprofit firms in a three-sector economy* (pp. 115–134). Washington, DC: The Urban Institute.

Hatry, H. P. (1983). *A review of private approaches for the delivery of public services.* Washington, DC: The Urban Institute Press.

Hauber, F. A., Bruininks, R. H., Hill, B. K., Lakin, K. C., & White, C. C. (1982). *National census of residential facilities: Fiscal year 1982.* Minneapolis, MN: University of Minnesota, Department of Educational Psychology.

Hayden, A. (1979). Handicapped children, birth to age 3. *Exceptional Children, 45,* 510–516.

"Health care spending: Can the rate of ascent be sowed?" (1981). *HCFA Forum Health Care Financing Review, 5*(3), 2–9.

Hill, B. K., Lakin, K. C., & Bruininks, R. H. (1984). *Trends in residential services for mentally retarded people 1977–1982.* Minneapolis, MN: University of Minnesota, Department of Educational Psychology.

Hill, M. & Wehman, P. (1983). Cost-benefit analysis of placing moderately and severely handicapped individuals into competitive employment. *TASH, 8*(1), 30–38.

Hofferbert, R. I. (1968). Socioeconomic dimensions of the American states: 1890–1960. *Midwest Journal of Political Science, 12,* 401–418.

Hofferbert, R. I. (1974). *The study of public policy.* Indianapolis, IN: Bobbs-Merrill.

Horejsi, C. R. (1979). Social and psychological factors in family care. In R. H. Bruininks & G. C. Krantz (Eds.), *Family care of developmentally disabled members: Conference proceedings* (pp. 13–24). Minneapolis, MN: University of Minnesota.

Howards, I., Brehm, H. P., & Nagi, S. Z. (1980). *Disability: From social problem to federal program.* New York: Praeger.

Human Services Research Institute (HSRI). (1985a). *The developmental disabilities strategic planning model.* Cambridge, MA: Author.

Human Services Research Institute. (1985b). *Services for persons with developmental disabilities: Standard definitions.* Boston, MA: Author.

Humm-Delgado, D. (1980). Planning issues in local interagency collaboration. In J. O. Elder & P. R. Magrab (Eds.), *Coordinating services to handicapped children: A handbook for interagency collaboration,* (pp. 163–178). Baltimore: Paul H. Brookes Publishing Co.

Hunt, R. C., & Wiley, E. D. (1968). Operation Baxstrom after one year. *American Journal of Psychiatry, 124,* 974–978.

Ilchman, W. F., & Upoff, N. T. (1969). *The political economy of change.* Berkeley, CA: University of California Press.

Intagliata, J. (1982). Improving the quality of community care for the chronically mentally disabled: The role of case management. *Schizophrenia Bulletin, 8*(4), 655–674.

Intagliata, J., Kraus, S., & Willer, B. (1980). The impact of deinstitutionalization on a community-based service system. *Mental Retardation, 18,* 305–307.

Janicki, M. P., Castellani, P. J., & Norris, R. G. (1983). Organization and administration of service delivery systems. In J. L. Matson & J. A. Mulick (Eds.), *Handbook of mental retardation* (pp. 3–23). New York: Pergamon.

Janicki, M. P., & Jacobson, J. W. (1986). Generational trends in sensory, physical and behavioral abilities among older mentally retarded persons. *American Journal of Mental Deficiency, 90*(5), 490–500.

Janicki, M. P., Krauss, M. W., Cotton, P. D., & Seltzer, M. M. (1986). Respite services and older adults with developmental disabilities. In C. L. Salisbury & J. Intagliata (Eds.), *Respite care: Support for persons with developmental disabilities and their families* (pp. 51–67). Baltimore: Paul H. Brookes Publishing Co.

Janicki, M. P., MacEachron, A. E. (1984). Residential, health and social service needs of elderly developmentally disabled persons. *The Gerontologist, 84,* 128–137.

Janicki, M. P., Otis, J. P., Puccio, P. S., Rettig, J. H., & Jacobson, J. W. (1985). Service needs among older developmentally disabled persons. In M. P. Janicki & H. M. Wisniewski (Eds.), *Aging and developmental disabilities: Issues and approaches* (pp. 289–304). Baltimore: Paul H. Brookes Publishing Co.

Janovsky, A., Scallet, L., & Jaskulski, T. (1983). *The county government role in mental health systems.* Washington, DC: National Association of Counties Research Inc.

Jaskulski, T. M., (1983a). *Issues affecting the county government role in mental health.* Washington, DC: National Association of Counties Research Inc.

Jaskulski, T. M. (1983b). *Trends in the county government role in mental health systems.* Washington, DC: National Association of Counties.

Jones, M. L., Hannah, J. K., Fawcett, A. B., Seekins, T., & Buddle, J. F. (1984). The independent living movement: A model for community integration of persons with disabilities. In W. P. Christian, G. Hannah, & T. J. Glahn (Eds.), *Programming effective human services.* New York: Plenum.

Justice, R. S., O'Connor, G., & Warren, W. (1971). Problems reported by parents of mentally retarded children: Who helps? *American Journal of Mental Deficiency, 75,* 685–691.

Kadushin, A. (1980). *Child welfare services* (3rd ed.) New York: Macmillan.

Kakalik, J. S., Fury, W. S., Thomas, M. A., & Carney, M. F. (1981). *The costs of special education: Summary of study findings.* Santa Monica, CA: The Rand Corp.

Kane, R. L., & Kane, R. A. (1978, May 6). Care of the aged: Old problems in need of new solutions. *Science,* pp. 913–919.

Keith, K. D., & Ferdinand, R. (1984). Changes in levels of mental retardation:

A comparison of institutional and community populations. *The Journal of the Association of Persons with Severe Handicaps, 9,* 26–30.

Kerachsky, S., Thornton, C., Bloomenthal, A., Maynard, R., & Stephens, S. (1985). *The impacts of transitional employment for mentally retarded young adults: Results from the STETS Demonstration.* New York: Manpower Demonstration Research Corporation.

Kernan, K. T., & Walker, M. W. (1981). Use of services for the mentally retarded in the African-American community. *Journal of Community Psychology, 9,* 45–52.

Kiernan, W. E. (1979). Rehabilitation planning. In P. R. Magrab & J. O. Elder (Eds.), *Planning for services to handicapped persons: Community, education, health* (pp. 137–171). Baltimore: Paul H. Brookes Publishing Co.

Kiernan, W. E., & Bruininks, R. H. (1986). Demographic characteristics. In W. E. Kiernan & J. A. Stark (Eds.), *Pathways to employment for adults with developmental disabilities* (pp. 21–50). Baltimore: Paul H. Brookes Publishing Co.

Kiernan, W. E., & Ciborowski, J., (1985). *Employment survey for adults with developmental disabilities.* Washington, DC: National Association of Rehabilitation Facilities.

Kiernan, W. E., Smith, B. C., & Ostrowsky, M. B. (1986). Developmental disabilities: Definitional issues. In W. E. Kiernan & J. A. Stark (Eds.), *Pathways to employment for adults with developmental disabilities* (pp. 11–20). Baltimore: Paul H. Brookes Publishing Co.

Kiernan, W. E. & Stark, J. A. (1986). Comprehensive design for the future. In W. E. Kiernan & J. A. Stark (Eds.), *Pathways to employment for adults with developmental disabilities* (pp. 103–111). Baltimore, MD. Paul H. Brookes Publishing Co.

Kimberly, J. R. (1968). *The financial structure of sheltered workshops.* Ithaca, NY: Region II Rehabilitation Research Institute, New York School of Industrial and Labor Relations, Cornell University.

Lakin, K. C., & Bruininks, R. H. (1985). Contemporary services for handicapped children and youth. In R. H. Bruininks and K. C. Lakin (Eds.), *Living and learning in the least restrictive environment* (pp. 3–22). Baltimore: Paul H. Brookes Publishing Co.

Lakin, K. C., & Hill, B. K. (1985). Target population. In K. C. Lakin, B. K. Hill, & R. H. Bruininks (Eds.), *An analysis of Medicaid's Intermediate Care Facility for the Mentally Retarded (ICF/MR) Program* (pp. 2-1–2-44). Minneapolis, MN: University of Minnesota, Department of Educational Psychology.

Lakin, K. C., Hill, B. K., & Bruininks, R. H. (Eds.). (1985). *An analysis of Medicaid's Intermediate Care Facility for the Mentally Retarded (ICF/MR) Program.* Minneapolis: University of Minnesota, Department of Educational Psychology.

Lakin, K. C., Hill, B. K., Bruininks, R. H., & White, C. C. (1986). Residential options and future implications. In W. E. Kiernan and J. A. Stark (Eds.), *Pathways to employment for adults with developmental disabilities* (pp. 207–228). Baltimore: Paul H. Brookes Publishing Co.

LaPorte, T. R. (1975). Organized social complexity: Explication of a concept. In T. R. LaPorte (Ed.), *Organized social complexity: Challenge to politics and policy* (pp. 3–21). Princeton, NJ: Princeton University Press.

Laski, F. J. (1985). Right to habilitation and right to education: The legal foundation. In R. H. Bruninks & K. C. Lakin (Eds.), *Living and learning in the least restrictive environment* (pp. 67–79). Baltimore: Paul H. Brookes Publishing Co.

Legislative Commission on Expenditure Review (New York State) (LCER). (1983). *Mental Health Community Support System.* Albany: Program Audit.

Legislative Commission on Expenditure Review (New York State) (LCER). (1984). *Family court orders for handicapped children.* Albany: Author.

Lessen, E., & Rose, T. (1980). State definitions of preschool handicapped populations. *Exceptional Children, 46,* 467–469.

Levitan, S., & Taggart, R. (1982). Rehabilitation, employment and the disabled. In J. Rubin & V. LaPorte (Eds.), *Alternatives in rehabilitating the handicapped: A policy analysis.* New York: Human Services Press.

Lindblom, C. E. (1977). *Politics and markets.* New York: Basic Books.

Lipset, S. M. (1959). Some social requisites of democracy: Economic development and political legitimacy. *American Political Science Review, 53,* 60–105.

Lowi, T. J. (1979). *The end of liberalism* (2nd ed.) New York: Norton.

Lubin, R., Jacobson, J. W., & Kiely, M. (1982). Projected impact of the functional definition of developmental disabilities: The categorical disabled population and service eligibility. *American Journal of Mental Deficiency, 87*(1), 73–79.

MacEachron, A. E. (1983). *Analysis of case management activities.* Albany: New York State Office of Mental Retardation and Developmental Disabilities.

MacEachron, A. E., Pensky, D., & Hawes, B. (1986). Case management for families of developmentally disabled clients: An empirical policy analysis of a statewide system. In J. J. Gallagher & P. M. Vietze (Eds.), *Families of handicapped persons: Research, programs, and policy issues* (pp. 273–287). Baltimore: Paul H. Brookes Publishing Co.

Meyers, C. E., Nihira, K., & Zetlin, A. (1979). The measurement of adaptive behavior. In N. Ellis (Ed.), *Handbook of mental deficiency* (2nd ed.) (pp. 431–481). Hillsdale, NJ: Lawrence Erlbaum Associates.

Meyers, W., (1985, November 24). The Nonprofits drop the 'non.' *New York Times,* p. B1.

Mills, v. D. C. Board of Education, 348 F. Supp 866 (D.D.C. 1972).

Minnesota Developmental Disabilities Program. (1982). *Policy analysis series paper no. 11: An analysis of Minnesota property values of community intermediate care facilities for mentally retarded (ICF-MRs).* St. Paul, MN: Developmental Disabilities Program, Department of Energy, Planning and Development.

Minnesota Developmental Disabilities Program. (1983). *Policy analysis series paper no. 18: The Minnesota Family Subsidy Program: Its effect on families with a developmentally disabled child.* St. Paul, MN: Developmental Disabilities Program, Department of Energy, Planning and Development.

Montgomery, J. (1982). The economics of supportive services for families with disabled and aging members. *Family Relations, 31,* 19–27.

Moroney, R. M. (1981). Mental disability: The role of the family. In J. J. Bevilacqua (Ed.), *Changing government policies for the mentally disabled* (pp. 209–238). Cambridge, MA: Ballinger Publishing Co.

Moroney, R. M. (1983). Families, care of the handicapped, and public policy. In R. Perlman (Ed.), *Family home care: Critical issues for services and policies* (pp. 188–212). New York: The Haworth Press.

Morrissey, J. P., Hall, R. H., & Lindsey, M. L. (1982). *Interorganizational relations: A sourcebook of measures for mental health programs.* Albany: New York State Office of Mental Health.

Nakamura, R. T., & Smallwood F. (1980). *The politics of implementation.* New York: St. Martin's Press.

Nathan, R., & Adams, C. (1976, Spring). Understanding central city hardship. *Political Science Quarterly, 91,* 47–62.

National Association of Rehabilitation Facilities. (1985). *From theory to implementation: A guide to supported employment for rehabilitation facilities.* Washington, DC: Author.

National Association of State Mental Retardation Program Directors (NASMRPD). (1979). *The minimal array of essential services for mentally retarded persons.* Alexandria, VA: Author.

National Association of State Mental Retardation Program Directors (NASMRPD). (1984). Critical issues surrounding the operation of Medicaid Home and Community Care Programs: An analysis based on interviews with MR/DD officials in selected states. Alexandria, VA: Author.

National Institute of Mental Health (NIMH). (1985). *Network analysis methods for mental health systems research: A comparison of two community support systems* (DHHS Pub. No. ADM 85-1383). Washington DC: U.S. Government Printing Office.

National Study Group on State Medicaid Strategies. (1983). *Restructuring Medicaid: An agenda for change.* Washington, DC: Center for the Study of Social Policy.

New York City Human Resources Administration. (1984). *The management of publicly financed home care.* New York: Author.

New York State. (1984). *Chapter 462, Laws of 1984.*

New York State Association for Retarded Children, Inc. (ARC). (1985). *Directory of chapters' programs and services.* Delmar, NY: Author.

New York State Association for Retarded Children and Parisi v. Rockefeller. 72 Civ. 356 (E. D. N. Y. 1972).

New York State Association for Retarded Children and Parisi v. Rockefeller. 72 Civ. 356 (E. D. N. Y. 1972). Memorandum, April 10, 1973.

New York State Association for Retarded Children and Parisi v. Rockefeller. 393 F. Supp. 715 (E. D. N. Y. 1975).

New York State Developmental Disabilities Planning Council. (1983). *Developmental disabilities plan of New York: 1984–1986.* Albany: Author.

New York State Education Department. (1985). *Service centers for independent living: Annual report.* Albany: Author.

New York State Governor's Select Commission on the Future of the State-Local Mental Health System. (1984). *Final report.* Albany: Author.

New York State Office of Mental Retardation and Developmental Disabilities (OMRDD). (1982). *Case management in the New York State Office of Mental Retardation and Developmental Disabilities: A report to the Commissioner.* Albany: Author.

New York State Office of Mental Retardation and Developmental Disabilities (OMRDD). (1983). *Local services project: The provision of planning of support services Phase I report.* Albany: Author.

New York State Office of Mental Retardation and Developmental Disabilities (OMRDD). (1985). *Summary of 1984–85 county local share.* Albany: Author.

Nirje, B. (1969). The principle of normalization and its human management implications. In R. Kugel & W. Wolfensberger (Eds.), *Changing patterns in residential services for the mentally retarded* (pp. 179–195). Washington, DC: U.S. Government Printing Office.

Noble, J. H., Jr. (1985, July). *The benefits and costs of supported employment and impediments to its expansion.* Paper presented at the Policy Seminar on Supported Employment, Virginia Institute for Developmental Disabilities, Virginia Commonwealth University, Richmond, VA.

Novak, A. R. (1980). Backlash to the deinstitutionalization movement. In A. R. Novak & L. W. Heal (Eds.), *Integration of developmentally disabled individuals into the community* (pp. 181–189). Baltimore: Paul H. Brookes Publishing Co.

Novak, A. R., & Heal, L. W. (Eds.). (1980). *Integration of developmentally disabled individuals into the community.* Baltimore: Paul H. Brookes Publishing Co.

O'Neill, J. H. (1984). *Analysis of starting salary parity between the New York State Office of Mental Retardation and Developmental Disabilities and United Cerebral Palsy Association of New York State.* New York: Author.

Oregon study revealed wage benefit differences for staff of publicly and privately operated facilities, (1985, June). *Links,* pp. 17–18.

Paine, S. C., Bellamy, G. T., & Wilcox, B. (1984). *Human services that work: From innovation to standard practice.* Baltimore: Paul H. Brookes Publishing Co.

Parker, R. A. (1985). Matching federal spending to need: An urban policy scorecard, 1977–1983. *Policy Studies Journal, 13,*(3), 625–633.

Parks, R. B., & Ostrom, E. (1981). Complex models of urban service systems. In T. N. Clark (Ed.), *Urban policy analysis: Directions for future research,* pp. 171–199). Beverly Hills, CA: Sage Publications.

Pennsylvania Association for Retarded Children v. Commonwealth of Pennsylvania, 343 F. Supp. 279 (1972).

Pepper, B. (1978). *The effects of state mental hygiene activities on Rockland County: Fiscal and programmatic impact.* Pomona, NY: A Report Prepared for the Legislature of Rockland County.

Perlman, R. (1983). Use of the tax system in home care: A brief note. In R. Perlman (Ed.), *Family home care: Critical issues for services and policies* (pp. 280–283). New York: Haworth Press.

Perlman, R. (1985). Family support options: A policy perspective. In J. M. Agosta & V. J. Bradley (Eds.), *Family care for persons with developmental disabilities: A growing commitment* (pp. 220–250). Boston: Human Services Research Institute.

Perlman, R., & Giele, J. Z. (1983). An unstable triad: Dependents' demands, family resources, community supports. In R. Perlman (Ed.), *Family home care: Critical issues for services and policies* (pp. 12–44). New York: Haworth Press.

Piachaud, D., Bradshaw, J., & Weale, J. (1981). The income effect of a disabled child. *Journal of Epidemiology and Community Health, 35,* 123–127.

President's Committee on Mental Retardation. (1977). *A national multi-*

cultural seminar on mental retardation among minority disadvantaged populations. Norfolk, VA: Author.

Pressman, J. L., & Wildavsky, A. (1973). *Implementation.* Berkeley: University of California Press.

Reif, M. E. (1985). *Analysis and recommendations regarding the administration and organization of the service delivery system in New York State for children with handicapping conditions under three years of age.* Rochester, NY. Regional Early Childhood Direction Center.

Rein, M., & Rabinowitz, F. F. (1978). Implementation: A theoretical perspective. In W. D. Burnham & M. W. Weinberg (Eds.), *American politics and public policy.* Cambridge, MA: MIT Press.

Reschly, D. J., & Jipson, F. J. (1976). Ethnicity, geographic locale, age, sex, and urban-rural residence as variables in the prevalence of mild retardation. *American Journal of Mental Deficiency, 18,* 154–161.

Rockowitz, R., & Davidson, P. (1986). *Developmentally disabled project: Final report.* Rochester, NY: University of Rochester, University Affiliated Program.

Rostow, W. W. (1964). *The stages of economic growth: A non-communist manifesto.* London: Cambridge University Press.

Rotegard, L. L., Bruininks, R. H., Holman, J. G., & Lakin, K. C. (1985). Environmental aspects of deinstitutionalization. In R. H. Bruininks & K. C. Lakin (Eds.), *Living and learning in the least restrictive environment* (pp. 155–184). Baltimore: Paul H. Brookes Publishing Co.

Roth, W. (1979). An economic model of social and psychological factors in families with developmentally disabled children. In R. H. Bruininks & G. C. Krantz (Eds.), *Family care of developmentally disabled members: Conference proceedings* (pp. 39–43). Minneapolis: University of Minnesota.

Rothman, D. (1971). *The discovery of the asylum: Social order and disorder in the new republic.* Boston: Little, Brown, & Co.

Rothman, D. J., & Rothman, S. M. (1984). *The Willowbrook wars.* New York: Harper & Row.

Rouse v. Cameron, 387 F. 2nd 241 (1967).

Rubin, J. (1978). *Economics, mental health and the law.* Lexington, MA: D.C. Heath.

Rubin, J. (Ed.) with LaPorte, V. (1982). *Alternatives in rehabilitating the handicapped: A policy analysis.* New York: Human Sciences Press.

Runkel, J. A. (1985). *Our childrens' voice.* Delmar: New York State Association for Retarded Children, Inc.

Ryan, S., & Coyne, A. (1985). Effects of group homes on neighborhood property values. *Mental Retardation, 23*(5), 241–245.

Sachs, M. L., Smull, M. W., & Beverely, B. K. (1985). *Selected demographic and need characteristics of respondents to the community needs survey for persons with non-retarded developmental disabilities.* Baltimore: University of Maryland School of Medicine.

Salamon, L. M., & Abramson, A. J. (1982). *The federal budget and the non-profit sector.* Washington, DC: The Urban Institute Press.

Savage, V. T., Novak, A. R., & Heal, L. W. (1980). Generic services for developmentally disabled citizens. In A. R. Novak & L. W. Heal (Eds.), *Integration of developmentally disabled individuals into the community* (pp. 75–89). Baltimore: Paul H. Brookes Publishing Co.

Schalock, R. L., & Keith, K. D. (1986). A resource allocation approach to determining a client's need status. *Mental Retardation, 28*(1), 27–35.

Scheerenberger, R. (1975). *Current trends and status of public residential services for the mentally retarded*. Madison, WI: National Association of Superintendents of Public Residential Facilities for the Mentally Retarded.

Schielke, D. (1984). *Overburden of excessive multiple fiscal reporting requirements*. Buffalo: United Cerebral Palsy Association of Western New York.

Schultze, W. A. (1985). *Urban politics: A political economy approach*. Englewood Cliffs, NJ: Prentice-Hall.

Seidl, F. W., Applebaum, R., Austin, C., & Mahoney, K. (1983). *Delivering in-home services to the aged and disabled*. Lexington, MA: Lexington Books.

Seltzer, M. M. (1985). Informal supports for elderly mentally retarded persons. *American Journal of Mental Deficiency, 89*, 257–266.

Seltzer, M. M., & Seltzer, G. B. (1985). The elderly mentally retarded: A group in need of service. *Journal of Gerontological Social Work, 8*, 99–119.

Sharkansky, I. (1967). Government expenditures and public policies in the American states. *American Political Science Review, 61*, 1066–1077.

Sharkansky, I. (1970). *The routines of politics*. New York: Van Nostrand Reinhold.

Shestakofsky, S., Van Gelder, M. M., & Kiernan, W. E. (1986). Evaluation, training, and placement in natural work environments. In W. E. Kiernan & J. A. Stark (Eds.), *Pathways to employment for adults with developmental disabilities* (pp. 185–197). Baltimore: Paul H. Brookes Publishing Co.

Shulman, D., & Galanter, R. (1976, Spring). Reorganizing the nursing home industry: A proposal. *Milbank Memorial Fund Quarterly*, pp. 129–143.

Sigelman, C. K., Novak, A. R., Heal, L. W., & Switzky, H. N. (1980). Factors that affect the success of community placement. In A. R. Novak & L. W. Heal (Eds.), *Integration of developmentally disabled individuals into the community* (pp. 57–74). Baltimore: Paul H. Brookes Publishing Co.

Simeonsson, R. J., & Bailey, D. B., Jr. (1986). Siblings of handicapped children. In J. J. Gallagher & P. M. Vietze (Eds.), *Families of handicapped persons: Research, programs, and policy issues* (pp. 67–77). Baltimore: Paul H. Brookes Publishing Co.

Smith, B. J. (1984). Expanding the federal role in serving young special-needs children. *Topics in Early Childhood Special Education, 4*(1), 33–42.

Special Committee to Study Commitment Procedures of the Association of the Bar of the City of New York. (1962). *Mental illness and due process: Report and recommendations on admissions to mental hospitals under New York law*. Ithaca, NY: Cornell University Press.

Spivey, W. A. (1985, May). Problems and paradoxes in economic and social policies of modern welfare states. *Annals of the American Academy of Political & Social Science, 479*, 14–30.

Staniland, M. (1985). *What is political economy: A study of social theory and underdevelopment*. New Haven, CT: Yale University Press.

Starr, P. (1978). Medicine and the waning of professional sovereignty. *Daedalus, 107*(1), 175–193.

Steadman, H. J., & Cocozza, J. J. (1974). *The careers of the criminally insane.* Lexington, MA: Lexington Books.

Stein, Z., & Susser M. (1975). Public health and mental retardation: new power and new problems. In M. J. Begab & S. A. Richardson (Eds.), *The mentally retarded and society: A social science perspective* (pp. 53–73). Baltimore: University Park Press.

Stoikov, V. (1970). Economics of scale in sheltered workshop operations. *Rehabilitation, sheltered workshops and the disadvantaged.* Ithaca, NY: Cornell University Press.

Stone, D. A. (1984). *The disabled state.* Philadelphia: Temple University Press.

Study Committee on Policy Management Assistance. (1975). *Strengthening public management in the intergovernmental system: A report prepared for the Office of Management and Budget.* Washington, DC: Author.

Sue, S., & McKinney, H. (1975). Asian Americans in the community mental health system. *American Journal of Orthopsychiatry, 43,* 111–118.

Summers, J. (1981). The definition of developmental disabilities: A concept in transition. *Mental Retardation, 19*(6), 259–265.

Sussman, M. (1982). Vocational rehabilitation for policy. In J. Rubin & V. LaPorte (Eds.), *Alternatives in rehabilitating the handicapped: A policy analysis.* New York: Human Sciences Press.

Szasz, T. (1963). *Law, liberty and psychiatry: An inquiry into the social uses of mental health practices.* New York: Collier Books.

Tausig, M. B., & Epple, W. A. (1985). *The placement process: Individual family and service factors.* Albany: New York State Office of Mental Retardation and Developmental Disabilities.

Thornton, C. (1985). Benefit-cost analysis of social programs: Deinstitutionalization and education programs. In R. H. Bruininks & K. C. Lakin (Eds.), *Living and learning in the least restrictive environment* (pp. 225–244). Baltimore: Paul H. Brookes Publishing Co.

Tjossem, T. (1976). Early intervention: Issues and approaches. In T. Tjossem (Ed.), *Intervention strategies for high risk and handicapped children.* Baltimore: University Park Press.

Turnbull, A. P., Brotherson, M. J., & Summers, J. A. (1985). The impact of deinstitutionalization on families: A family systems approach. In R. H. Bruininks & K. C. Lakin (Eds.), *Living and learning in the least restrictive environment* (pp. 115–140). Baltimore: Paul H. Brookes Publishing Co.

Turnbull, A. P., Summers, J. A., & Brotherson, M. J. (1986). Family life cycle: Theoretical and empirical implications and future directions for families with mentally retarded members. In J. J. Gallagher & P. M. Vietze (Eds.), *Families of handicapped persons: Research, programs, and policy issues* (pp. 45–65). Baltimore, Paul H. Brookes Publishing Co.

United States Department of Health and Human Services. (1981). *The developmental disabilities movement: A national study of minority participation.* Washington, DC: Author.

United States Small Business Administration (1984). *Unfair competition by nonprofit organizations with small business: An issue for the 1980's.* Washington, DC: Author.

Vandernoot, J. (1984). Analysis of fiscal years and reporting requirements. Westchester ARC, White Plains, NY. Unpublished manuscript.

Wehman, P. (1981). *Competitive employment: New horizons for severely disabled individuals*. Baltimore: Paul H. Brookes Publishing Co.

Wehman, P., & Kregel, J. (1985). A supported work approach to competitive employment of persons with moderate and severe handicaps. *Journal of the Association for the Severely Handicapped, 10*(1), 3–11.

Wehman, P. H., Kregel, J., Barcus, J. M., & Schalock, R. L. (1986). Vocational transition for students with developmental disabilities. In W. E. Kiernan & J. A. Stark (Eds.), *Pathways to employment for adults with developmental disabilities* (pp. 113–127). Baltimore: Paul H. Brookes Publishing Co.

Weisbrod, B. A. (1975). Toward a theory of the voluntary nonprofit sector in a three sector economy. In E. Phelps (Ed.) *Altruism, morality and economic theory*. New York: Russell Sage Foundation.

Weisbrod, B. A. (1977). *The voluntary nonprofit sector*. Lexington, MA: Lexington Books.

Welch, G. T. (1982). Private and public rehabilitation. In J. Rubin & V. LaPorte (Eds.), *Alternatives in rehabilitating the handicapped: A policy analysis*. New York: Human Sciences Press.

White, M. J. (Ed.). (1981a). *Nonprofit firms in a three sector economy*. Washington, DC: The Urban Institute Press.

White, M. J. (1981b). An introduction to the nonprofit sector. In M. J. White (Ed.), *Nonprofit firms in a three sector economy* (pp. 1–9). Washington, DC: The Urban Institute Press.

Wieck, C. A. (1980). *The cost of public and community residential care for mentally retarded people in the United States* (unpublished doctoral dissertation, University of Minnesota, 1980)

Wieck, C. A. (1985). The development of family support programs. In J. M. Agosta & V. J. Bradley (Eds.), *Family care for persons with developmental disabilities: A growing commitment* (pp. 70–93). Boston: Human Services Research Institute.

Wieck, C. A., & Bruininks, R. H. (1981). *The cost of public and community residential care for the mentally retarded people in the United States*. Minneapolis, MN: University of Minnesota, Department of Educational Psychology.

Wieck, K. E. (1976). Educational organizations as loosely coupled systems. *Administrative Science Quarterly, 21*, 1–9.

Wikler, L. M. (1986). Family stress theory and research on families of children with mental retardation. In J. J. Gallagher & P. M. Vietze (Eds.) *Families of handicapped persons: Research, programs, and policy issues* (pp. 167–195). Baltimore: Paul H. Brookes Publishing Co.

Wisniewski, K., & Hill, A. L. (1985). Clinical aspects of dementia in mental retardation and developmental disabilities. In M. P. Janicki & H. M. Wisniewski (Eds.), *Aging and developmental disabilities: Issues and approaches* (pp. 195–206). Baltimore: Paul H. Brookes Publishing Co.

Wolfensberger, W. (1972). *The principle of normalization in human services*. Toronto: National Institute on Mental Retardation.

Wolfensberger, W. (1983). Social role valorization: A proposed new term for the principle of normalization: *Mental Retardation, 21*(6), 234–239.

Wolfensberger, W., & Glenn, L. (1973). *Program analysis of service systems (PASS): A method for the quantitative evaluation of human services: Handbook*. Toronto: National Institute on Mental Retardation.

Wolfensberger, W., & Thomas S. (1983). *Passing program analysis of service systems' implementation of normalization goals: Normalization criteria and ratings manual* (2nd ed.). Downsview, Ontario: National Institute on Mental Retardation.

Wolfensberger, W., & Tullman, S. (1982). A brief outline of the principle of normalization. *Rehabilitation Psychology, 27*(3), 131–145.

Wolpert, J. (1978). *Group homes for the mentally retarded: An investigation of neighborhood property impacts.* Princeton, NJ: Princeton University Press.

Wyatt v. Stickney, 344 F. Supp. 387 (M.D. Ala 1972).

Young, D. R. (1981). Entrepreneurship and the behavior of nonprofit organizations: Elements of a theory. In M. J. White (Ed.), *Nonprofit firms in a three sector economy* (pp. 135–162). Washington, DC: The Urban Institute Press.

Zeller, R. W. (1980). Direction service: Collaboration one case at a time. In J. O. Elder & P. R. Magrab (Eds.), *Coordinating services to handicapped children: A handbook for interagency collaboration* (pp. 65–97). Baltimore: Paul H. Brookes Publishing Co.

Zimmerman, S. L. (1984). The mental retardation family subsidy program: Its effects on families with a mentally handicapped child *Family Relations,* pp. 105–118.

Zuckerman, H. S. (1983). Industrial rationalization of a contract industry: Multi-institutional hospital systems. *Annals of the American Academy of Political and Social Sciences, 468,* 216–230.

Index